ENDURANCE

How Faith Can Help You Win the Race

Thomas D. Logie

Order this book online at www.trafford.com
or email orders@trafford.com

Most Trafford titles are also available at major online book retailers.

© Copyright 2010 Thomas D. Logie.
All rights reserved. No part of this publication may be reproduced, stored in a retrieval system, or transmitted, in any form or by any means, electronic, mechanical, photocopying, recording, or otherwise, without the written prior permission of the author.

Printed in Victoria, BC, Canada.

ISBN: 978-1-4269-2941-0 (sc)
ISBN: 978-1-4269-2942-7 (e-book)

Our mission is to efficiently provide the world's finest, most comprehensive book publishing service, enabling every author to experience success. To find out how to publish your book, your way, and have it available worldwide, visit us online at www.trafford.com

Trafford rev. 4/30/2010

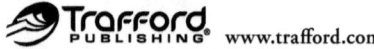 www.trafford.com

North America & international
toll-free: 1 888 232 4444 (USA & Canada)
phone: 250 383 6864 ♦ fax: 812 355 4082

AN INTRODUCTORY NOTE ON SHADES OF MEANING

Our central subject is Christian endurance. Closely allied to endurance are patience and perseverance. Patience is the ability to endure delay without complaint. Many of us have had to be patient when airplanes or other conveyances of transport are delayed. It is not pleasant.

Endurance can be passive when trouble cannot be escaped. An anvil is a physical example of passive endurance. In pre-industrial days, how many hammers and hammers' handles were broken on a single anvil? Consider recent history. Three of the worst persecutors of Biblical Christianity were Hitler, Stalin and Mao Tse-tung. They are all dead. What of Christianity? In China, Russia and the Eastern European countries dominated by Stalin after World War 2, Christianity is especially resurgent even though still persecuted officially in China. There is still a Christian witness in Germany long after Naziism has been ruined.

There is another form of endurance known physically to the athlete and the soldier. With exertion, physical or spiritual, comes weariness and pain. This form of endurance allows a person to carry on in his or her duties (physical, family or other duties) despite the pain and the temptation to quit. As a boy, David knew this form of endurance as a shepherd living outdoors constantly in all weather. James Herriot, the author of <u>All Things Great and Small</u>, thought that the Yorkshire shepherds whom he knew were the most physically fit men he had seen. Such people are not passive in the way that an anvil is passive or in the manner that a Christian may be forced to physical passivity (or at least confined to a narrow scope of activity) by imprisonment for his or her faith. They are active in pursuing a duty despite obstacles and discomfort and grow strong in the process.

I would understand perseverance as being a pattern of continued active endurance. William Wilberforce, the British member of Parliament who spent his political life driving for and finally succeeding in abolishing slavery in the British Empire, is an example of perseverance. Winston Churchill is a 20th-century example of perseverance in rousing Great Britain from political slumber to wake up to the Hitler menace from 1933 into 1939. The Apostle Paul is another example for the work of Jesus Christ. Consider the list of his physical hardships up to the time he wrote 2 Corinthians 11:24-27:

> *Of the Jews five times received I thirty-nine stripes. Three times was I beaten with rods, once was I stoned, three times I suffered shipwreck, a night and a day I have been in the deep; in journeyings often, in perils of waters, in perils of robbers, in perils by mine own countrymen, in perils by the heathen, in perils in the city, in perils in the wilderness, in perils in the sea, in perils among false brethren; in weariness and painfulness, in watchings often, in hunger and thirst, in fastings often, in cold and nakedness.*

Paul must have been "one tough cookie" to have survived all this, but he did not proceed primarily in human strength. His own testimony is that *"I can do all things through Christ Who strengthens me."* Philippians 4:13. Through the strength that Jesus Christ gave him Paul perservered.

Often in this book I may use the term endurance where patience, both types of endurance and perseverance are all in mind. In wrestling with precise terminology I am not alone. Consider several public domain translations of Hebrews 10:36, which I will quote first in the King James Version: *For you have need of patience, that, after ye have done the will of God, ye might receive the promise.* John Nelson Darby used the word "endurance" where the King James translators used "patience." So does the Modern King James Version, which version I will use in this book unless otherwise specified. The Weymouth translation uses "patient endurance." The New King James translation substitutes "perseverance" for "patience" in several New Testament passages such as 2 Peter 1:6, James 5:11 and Romans 5:3-4. In truth we need patience, endurance and perseverance.

CHAPTER 1

THE NECESSITY OF ENDURANCE: GENERAL CONSIDERATIONS

God does not give us all the same race to run. We are commanded to *"run with endurance the race that is set before us."* Hebrews 12:1. Some, like the repentant robber on the cross on Golgotha next to our Lord Jesus, run a short sprint. That robber was saved a few hours before physical death and then entered Paradise with the Lord Jesus. In that brief time he left behind a timeless witness. Luke 23:39-43. Some children die young in faith. David Brainerd lived a relatively short life but full of prayer and efforts to reach lost souls. Many missionaries have died young either from disease or from violence from people who refused their message.

Others are given a figurative marathon or even an ultra-marathon to run. An attorney from a neighboring county to my own office has had the experience of running/walking 100 miles with a time limit of 24 hours. Of course special physical training is required to undertake such an effort. In the spiritual realm, consider Polycarp, believed to have been a convert to Jesus Christ under the ministry of the Apostle John. He was burned at the stake for his faith. When he was about to be burned Polycarp is reported to have said that "For 86 years I have served Christ and He has done me no wrong." We are not sure whether Polycarp was referring to his age on earth or to the years since his conversion, but in either case Polycarp was completing a very long race with a hard, uphill finish. In our own day Billy Graham has lived an extraordinarily long and faithful life. He must be in the closing stages of his marathon.

The prophet Daniel also lived an extraordinarily long life, extending from the initial capture of Jerusalem by the Babylonians (estimated at 605 B.C.) past the first return of the Jewish Captivity (approximately 535 B.C.) to at least "the third year of Cyrus" noted in Daniel 10:1. In all probability Daniel was at least 8 years old when he was taken captive to Babylon. Since Daniel had spent 70 years in Babylonian captivity before the capture of the Babylonian Empire by the Medes and Persians, he was at a minimum 80 years old when he received the vision started in Daniel 10. Daniel lived for some time serving under Darius, who handled the internal affairs of the early Persian empire while Cyrus was expanding it militarily. So Daniel could easily have been in his eighties when serving under Darius and nearly 90 when he died. This is certainly a marathon life with a stint in the Den of Lions when past 80.

As a final example, consider John the Apostle, the youngest of the original Twelve. When one reads the three letters written by John, they show grandfatherly tenderness, indicating that at least these were written when John was an old man. He had endured exile on Patmos. Historical reports which do not have the infallibility of Scripture claim that John was thrown into a vat of boiling oil but was not harmed by miracle. On this line of thought, John was exiled because the Romans could not carry out their death sentence. Much earlier, the Lord Jesus had told Peter (John 21:20-23) to follow Him even if John would not die. Some in the church interpreted this as a prophecy that John was not pass through death. John himself was careful to note that our Lord Jesus did not promise that he would not die. The Scriptures give no hint as to whether John died or how he departed this life. Other historical writings do not explain either. Perhaps John entered the presence of the Lord Jesus as a very old man without death, like Enoch or Elijah. We do know that John outlived all of the other Apostles and that a reasonable guess of his life span would be close to 85 years even if John was an older teenager when our Lord was crucified. His life could easily have been longer than this. When one considers the Gospel of John and Revelation in addition to the three short letters, John ran a marathon course or more.

We know from modern medical research that training for a sprint is quite different from training for long-distance running. Evander Holyfield and his trainers pioneered in specialized training for boxing, which in essence was composed of 10, 12 or 15 (in former days) windsprints with short rests in between. Derek Jeter changed his training methods before the 2009 baseball season to make his first moves more explosive. It worked. Track and field runners train explosively for sprints and finishing "kicks" and for cardiovascular training for distance. If God trains us differently from someone else, this is no cause for complaint. We may feel that God is being too hard on us. No, God is training us for our race and not for the race that another believer may have to run. The physical analogy is appropriate. Hebrews 12:5-7 says this:

> *And you have forgotten the exhortation which speaks to you as to sons: "My son, do not despise the chastening of the Lord, nor be discouraged when you are rebuked by Him; For whom the Lord loves He chastens, and scourges every son whom He receives." If you endure chastening, God deals with you as with sons; for what son is there whom a father does not chasten?*

In this vein also consider 1 Corinthians 9:24-27:

> *Do you not know that those who run in a race all run, but one receives the prize? Run in such a way that you may obtain it. And everyone who competes for the prize is temperate in all things. Now they do it to obtain a perishable crown, but we for an imperishable crown. Therefore I run thus: not with uncertainty. Thus I fight: not as one who beats the air. But I discipline my body and bring it into subjection, lest, when I have preached to others, I myself should become disqualified.*

In general, the more intense the training, the greater the ultimate prize and the more potential the trainer sees in the athlete.

Peter is an example of the principle that the trainer/discipler is hardest on the one who eventually can be greatest. While our Lord Jesus rebuked all of the disciples, only to Peter did he say, *"Get behind me, Satan!"* Matthew 16:23. Jesus was similarly severe on Peter concerning Peter's denials of our Lord, when all of the disciples were cowards to a lesser or greater extent. Our Lord Jesus was then tender with Peter in restoring him to his place as a leader among the disciples in John 21:15-23. If God is being hard with you, do not get angry with Him or try to drop out of the hard training He has appointed for you. Do not faint. Hebrews 12:5. Although this is hard, we need to give thanks that God is willing to spend His time in chastening and training us for His work despite our sin. Family discipline is a sign of membership in the family; its absence is a sign that we are not saved at all and are at immediate risk of everlasting judgment. Hebrews 12:5-13. The entire chapter of Hebrews 12 teaches the necessity of endurance in order to complete successive segments of God's continuous training for our good.

One further example of the necessity of physical and spiritual endurance will illustrate the point. Jacob and Isaac both dug wells. At Sychar our Lord Jesus drank from Jacob's well and converted the woman who had had five husbands and was "shacking up" with man #6. (John 4:5-6 refers to Jacob's well and the remainder of the chapter shows how our Lord saved the woman. Many more people were saved in Sychar when our Lord Jesus visited.) Isaac dug several wells in southern Israel (Genesis 26:15-33). In modern times we are prone to assume that good drinking water is here for the taking. I remember when my wife and I were building a house on a mountain lot that the well driller reached 10 gallons per minute at 200 feet. The whole process took a few hours. In the days of Jacob and Isaac this was not true. I do not know how deep any of these wells were, but we know that Jacob and Isaac had no machines to dig them. Bronze shovels would have been respectable technology for the day. Iron (let alone steel or aluminum) was not yet commonly available. Even allowing for the presence of servants with Isaac, digging even one of these wells would have been a considerable undertaking. There was presumably no other water in the vicinity, so the men would have had to return to a safe drinking water source already in existence. The loosened soil would have to be removed, and this process became more difficult as the well deepened. The side walls would have to be banked or kept secure in some way, along with a path to the water that a woman could walk. I do not know the soil characteristics, but from my experience of planting trees in Virginia clay a depth of 2 feet per person per hour would be an excellent rate of digging. If the depth were to be 200 feet as in my case, reaching water would take almost 2 weeks if one could dig for 8 hours a day with one person digging. The presence of servants might speed up the work, but some of them would have to be engaged in removing the soil and shoring walls instead of digging. My calculations are not precise, but are meant to give a sense of the reality behind the simple Biblical statements about wells being dug.

Let us connect this with endurance, particularly with the climate in Israel. It gets quite hot there in the summer. (Tel Aviv is about as far north as Savannah, Georgia.) Now let's imagine for a moment that your family needs a new well and you can get to a digging site and start digging an hour after sunrise. The temperature might be comfortable for the first hour or so. You can hope that the bugs won't be too bad. You can trust that you will not provoke any poisonous snakes. But the temperature rises and the sweat pours. There's no water in the area, but you try to keep digging into the heat of the day. Presumably you have some food and a skin of some kind of drink at lunch. Then it's back to digging again as the temperature rises even higher. You had better be sweating like a pig because you would be dehydrated if you aren't sweating. You might get heatstroke or sunstroke. If not, you stop exhausted and go back to your camp near a water source. But there's probably no water for a bath and any animals that you have need water too. Now imagine that you have put in 10 days' work and all you see is a hole in the ground. Do you stop on the idea that there is no water here? If you stop here and pick another dry hole you might be digging for almost a month with no results. Do you keep going on the theory that the water is just below you? If you stop too soon all of your effort has been wasted. Continuing is great if you're right, but ...

Digging these wells took endurance. Isaac knew some well sites from his time with his father Abraham, so at least his risk of a dry hole was less. He and his servants still had to unplug his father's wells and then settle differences with Abimelech. Building a spiritual life and a spiritual family takes spiritual endurance. In more recent times, financial endurance is often as necessary as physical endurance. We have read of "bridges to nowhere" where funding has been stopped in the middle of a project. A major commercial firm just surrendered a huge apartment complex in New

York to the lenders. Our Lord Jesus' question in Luke 14:28-30 concerning the tower sounds as if it came from last week's newspaper:

> *For which of you, intending to build a tower, does not sit down first and count the cost, whether he has enough to finish it; lest, after he has laid the foundation, and is not able to finish, all who see it begin to mock him, saying, 'This man began to build and was not able to finish.'*

So we can learn endurance by observing finance as well as physical labor. Debt supplies capital but also reduces financial endurance because of the drag of the debt repayments. Spiritually, because we have the riches of the Lord Jesus, we will have sufficient resources (spiritual especially, and secondarily financial and physical) to accomplish what He has called us to do. Ephesians 1:7 says that *"In Him we have redemption through His blood, the forgiveness of sins, according to the riches of His grace."* We are promised in Philippians 4:19 that *"My God shall supply all your need according to His riches in glory by Christ Jesus."* Sometimes we may misunderstand what God is calling us to do and need correction to get on the right track. Once we are headed in the right direction, we need endurance to continue to draw upon His grace until the task has been accomplished.

CHAPTER 2

NECESSITY OF ENDURANCE: EVIDENCE OF GENUINE CONVERSION

The Parable of the Soils (often called the Parable of the Sower) in Matthew 13 is a pivotal teaching of the Lord Jesus concerning His true Church and ministry. Read it carefully. For quick and convenient reference, I will try to compress the basics into a table:

Soil Type	Start	Root Type	Finish	Fruitfulness
Walking path	Seed on surface	None	Birds ate	None
Stony layer	Abundant foliage	Shallow	Scorched, dead	None
Thorny ground	Normal at first	Insufficient	Stunted, dead	None
Good ground	Normal growth	Deep	Maturity	**Abundant**

It is commonly hoped that the last three soils represent varieties of people who will be saved and reach heaven. When we read the parable carefully and compare other Scriptures, such hope is a delusion. Only the last soil is called good, and only the last soil yields a crop.

Since the hard, evil character of the hardpacked soil is so obvious, little time need be spent. Like so many people today, these people have hearts so hard that nothing can take root. In modern times, the comparable figure might be a highway or sidewalk. Satan acted in Jesus' day and so acts today to get the Word out of the minds of such people as rapidly as possible. Satan uses many distractions ranging from mind-distorting drugs to lewd entertainment to sarcastic denunciation of the Scriptures to overwork, among others. Such methods correspond to the birds of the air in the parable.

The stony ground is not merely ground with stones mixed in. What is described is ground with a very thin layer of topsoil with a solid layer of shale or other rock just beneath the surface. Such a rock layer cannot be removed by normal methods of agriculture. Grain cannot penetrate this solid layer. The result is abundant foliage immediately in the springtime because the energy that should be building solid roots is being redirected to the path of least resistance. But as the weather warms and the spring rains stop, the stunted roots cannot get water to sustain the foliage. The plant dies with no harvest.

The stony ground hearer may well believe the Word given at a surface level for the sake of the friendship and fellowship. In Matthew 13:21, it is persecution that drives this type of person away from the truth. Because of the lack of deep roots, this person leans on others for support and falls when external forces withdraw that support. Contrast this to the Apostle Paul, who said, *"Let God be true but every man a liar."* Romans 3:4. Paul stressed the knowledge of Jesus Christ person-to-person as the vital heart of Christianity. If friends fail, Jesus remains. Part of Paul's great ambition was to *"know Him, and the power of His resurrection, and the fellowship of His sufferings, being conformed to His death ..."* Philippians 3:10. In contrast to the person corresponding to the stony ground, our primary support must be Jesus Christ instead of other people. Paul rightly valued friendship and fellowship in Christ, but not as his primary source of life, joy or hope. Since Paul knew Jesus Christ personally, all other relationships (and for those of us who are married, even our relationships to our mates – see Matthew 19:29) were secondary to the one supreme relationship with Jesus Christ.

To compare, our Lord Jesus Himself taught that without knowing Him it is impossible to enter the Kingdom. Matthew 7:23.

Does the stony ground in the parable represent people who will be in heaven? Consider Matthew 24:9-13. Our Lord Jesus in teaching about the final days of history said this:

> *Then they will deliver you up to tribulation and kill you, and you will be hated by all nations for My name's sake. And then many will be offended, will betray one another, and will hate one another. Then many false prophets will rise up and deceive many. And because lawlessness will abound, the love of many [literally, the love of the many, i.e. the majority] will grow cold.* ***But he who endures to the end shall be saved.*** *(emphasis added)*

In comparing the two teachings by our Lord, the description of the love of the many growing cold corresponds to the people be offended who are represented by the stony ground. The "lawlessness" in Matthew 24:12 fits well with the "tribulation or persecution" of Matthew 13:21. Notice that the characteristic of the saved in Matthew 24:13 is endurance. Since the people represented by the stony ground lack endurance, they must be understood to be lost and doomed.

Further confirmation can be found near the close of the Sermon on the Mount. One clue is found in Matthew 7:13-14, which reads, *"Enter by the narrow gate; for wide is the gate and broad is the way that leads to destruction, and there are many who go in by it. Because narrow is the gate and difficult is the way which leads to life, and there are few who find it."* Our Lord is clear that only a relatively small minority of people living to maturity find the way to eternal life. That corresponds to the reading of the Parable of the Soils that only one of the four types of soils represents people who reach heaven.

The next section of the Sermon on the Mount (Matthew 7:16-20 – emphasis is added to verses 19-20) clinches the case. Our Lord said,

> *You will know them by their fruits. Do men gather grapes from thornbushes or figs from thistles? Even so, every good tree bears good*

> *fruit, but a bad tree bears bad fruit. A good tree cannot bear bad fruit, nor can a bad tree bear good fruit.* **Every tree that does not bear good fruit is cut down and thrown into the fire. Therefore by their fruits you will know them.**

In this sermon, the Lord Jesus teaches that only the fruitful shall escape the fire, which should ultimately be understood to be the Lake of Fire of Revelation. (John the Baptist taught the same thing as recorded in Luke 3:7-9.) John 15:5-6 also contrasts the branch that abides in Christ that bears fruit and the branch of the grapevine that does not abide in Christ and consequently bears no fruit. The fruitless are thrown into the fire and burned. While it seems hard at first reading, let us submit to the Lord Jesus and take Him at His Word. While we can perceive a difference between those who may cease bearing fruit because of physical weakness, advanced age and similar causes and those who have never borne fruit, we need to recognize that those who have never borne fruit are unconverted and doomed unless they repent and are granted eternal life by grace through faith. Particularly with the people represented by the stony ground and who "receive the word with joy" at first, our Lord's warning of Matthew 7:21 must be heard: *"Not everyone who says to Me, 'Lord, Lord,' shall enter the kingdom of heaven, but he who does the will of My Father in heaven."* In Matthew 7:22-23 such people attempt to cite alleged good works in the name of Christ, but He summarily rejects their claims because He never knew them. Additionally, there was no fruit as we know from the parable.

The thorny ground hearer represents the competition in the soul between Jesus Christ and the riches and concerns of this life. In this ground, earthly concerns prevail over the concerns of the Kingdom of Heaven. Since there is no fruit from this type of soil either, the people represented here also end up lost and doomed. In addition to the verses we just viewed on the necessity of fruitfulness, our Lord gave several illustrations about how riches and the concerns of this life, though valid in a subordinate place, can and do choke the spiritual life of the soul. Riches are not inherently wrong. Paul gave instructions to the believing rich in 1 Timothy 6:17-19 to trust God, avoid pride and to share. Both Joseph of Arimathea and Nicodemus, who honored the Lord Jesus publicly by attending to His body after His death on the Cross, were rich men. So was Job. But riches are dangerous, like explosive cargo which is indeed necessary but must be handled with great care. For the vast majority the prayer of Proverbs 30:7-9 is appropriate, and likewise the section of our Lord's Prayer which asks God for our daily bread.

I can give 3 Biblical examples of rich men who were strangled spiritually by their riches. One is found in Luke 16:19-31. We are not told how this man obtained his riches, but we do know that he dressed in excellent clothes and had a banquet every day. The beggar Lazarus sat at his gate for what scraps or alms he might get. The Scriptures do not say what notice the rich man took of Lazarus, but from the silence I would infer that this rich man ignored Lazarus. They both died about the same time. Once again the Scriptures do not say, but Lazarus probably died from the effects of extreme poverty and the rich man died from one of the diseases of wealth – a heart attack brought on by lavish eating is a reasonable inference. Lazarus died in faith and was comforted in the presence of Abraham (this is prior to the death and resurrection of Christ). The rich man died, and to his horror was tormented and found his tongue on fire. He who was so wealthy on earth now did not even have water! He never will again. Here is one man in whom riches choked all spiritual growth. The most he could desire was that someone could be sent to warn his brothers who were still living. In fact our Lord Jesus was sent to them as to all the house of Israel. But if the brothers would not hear and heed the words of Moses and the prophets, then they would not heed the Lord Jesus either even though He would and in fact did rise from the dead. We do not know what happened to the brothers, but for this rich man there was no mercy. What he was suffering in his holding place is but a fraction of what he and others like him will suffer in the Lake of Fire.

Then consider the case of the wealthy farmer, which the Lord Jesus described in a parable in Luke 12:16-21. Since this is a parable, there was no one particular farmer whom our Lord was describing, but the man was representative of many wealthy people. In this case we know that he had fertile soil and was a superior farmer. So his money was earned legitimately in terms of the commercial world. There are no accusations of false balances or other fraudulent methods. (Compare Proverbs 11:1; 16:11,

20:10, 23) The issue is not with the man's prosperity. In fact he was doing a good service to his neighbors by his farming, and God left the man alone so long as he was fulfilling his God-given purpose in an economic sense. The deadly problem is that the concerns of farming and riches had crowded out God Himself in the man's life, just as the thorns crowded out the good seed in the Parable of the Soils. When he decided to retire, he concentrated on his own comfort instead of serving his neighbors by his production. But the biggest problem is that there was no worship of God, which persisted throughout his work and marked his one-day retirement before his death. He had plenty of treasure on earth to take care of himself, but he had no riches in heaven. By contrast, our Lord Jesus said in an earlier portion of the Sermon on the Mount (Matthew 6:19-21, 24-34):

> *Do not lay up for yourselves treasures on earth, where moth and rust destroy and where thieves break in and steal; but lay up for yourselves treasures in heaven, where neither moth nor rust destroys and where thieves do not break in and steal. For where your treasure is, there your heart will be also.*
>
> *No one can serve two masters; for either he will hate the one and love the other, or else he will be loyal to the one and despise the other. You cannot serve God and mammon. Therefore I say to you, do not worry about your life, what you will eat or what you will drink; nor about your body, what you will put on. Is not life more than food and the body more than clothing? Look at the birds of the air, for they neither sow nor reap nor gather into barns; yet your heavenly Father feeds them. Are you not of more value than they? Which of you by worrying can add one cubit to his stature?*
>
> *So why do you worry about clothing? Consider the lilies of the field, how they grow: they neither toil nor spin, and yet I say to you that even Solomon in all his glory was not arrayed like one of these. Now if God so clothes the grass of the field, which today is, and tomorrow is thrown into the oven, will He not much more clothe you, O you of little faith?*

> *Therefore do not worry, saying, 'What shall we eat?' or 'What shall we drink?' or 'What shall we wear?' For after all these things the Gentiles seek. For your heavenly Father knows that you need all these things. But seek first the kingdom of God and His righteousness, and all these things shall be added to you. Therefore do not worry about tomorrow, for tomorrow will worry about its own things. Sufficient for the day is its own trouble.*

People represented by the thorny ground violate this warning and are traveling the broad way that leads to destruction as surely as the people represented by the rocky soil.

The man commonly known as the rich young ruler (Luke 18:18-27, also Mark 10:17-27) presents a more appealing picture than our previous two examples, but he also faced a struggle between following Jesus Christ and clinging to his possessions. This ruler came running to Jesus. His question was urgent and he was going to the right Man. He knew enough to call Jesus "good", in contrast to many of his contemporaries among the wealthy. He was humble enough to kneel before Jesus, confessing His superiority by gesture and perhaps even implying recognition as King of Israel. Mark says that Jesus "loved" him and that out of His love He commanded the man to give up his possessions. Jesus knew that the young man was in trouble with the Tenth Commandment even though he had at least outwardly observed the others. In this respect this young man was similar to Saul of Tarsus as a youth, who described himself as "blameless" concerning the righteousness of the Law (Philippians 3:6) but also covetous (Romans 7:7-11). The young man was sad when he heard what our Lord Jesus said. Would the cares of riches crowd out spiritual concerns in this man's case also? We are not told the end of the story.

What we can perceive from this incident is that covetousness is so deadly that extreme measures must be taken to uproot it. If necessary, all possessions not necessary to life have to be given up to crush it. Francis of Assisi centuries later made this very choice. Eric Liddell, portrayed in *Chariots of Fire,* made a similar choice to serve as a missionary in China when he could have been wealthy in England after the 1924 Olympics. What assets we do have we hold at God's pleasure. They are His to take away at any time. This is completely contrary to the mentality of those represented by the thorny ground. If such people remain as they are, they too are lost and doomed. Those whom God permits to have wealth are accountable to Him for how they are used and must remember that their assets belong to God and not to themselves.

The final soil in the Parable of the Soils is the good ground. The grain there takes root, endures the entire growing season and then produces an abundant crop. People represented by this ground show two necessary attributes of the saved and transformed people of God: **endurance** (for whatever time God should require) and **fruitfulness**.

Friend, if you are failing these tests of everlasting life, please pause right here and ask the Lord Jesus for His mercy to change you into good ground for His Word. You cannot change yourself, but He can change you as He has changed millions before. This is something He delights to do for anyone who asks honestly. The rich young ruler asked for an honest answer and received it as it applied to him. Let Him search all the recesses of your soul and plead with Him to start changing yours. Our Lord Jesus has changed a variety of people. Zacchaeus (Luke 19:1-10) was a shady tax collector. The woman at the well (John 4) was immoral. Legion (Mark 5:1-20; Luke 8:27-39) was demented to the point of living among the tombs in a cemetery. Nicodemus was a religious teacher (John 3:1-21). The Apostle Paul (Acts 9) was a determined persecutor of people now called Christians. If you look at 1 Corinthians 6:9-11, you will find a catalog of some of the sleaziest people who were saved and changed there. He can change you too, and you will grow to love the change.

CHAPTER 3

WHAT IS MEANT BY THE INCREASE IN THE PARABLE OF THE SOILS?

Matthew 13 and Mark 4 are not specific as to the type of seed sown in terms of physical crops. But we do know from nature that any type of sown seed that reaches maturity produces a crop like the original seed. As our Lord Jesus said in Matthew 7:16-17: *You will know them by their fruits. Do men gather grapes from thornbushes or figs from thistles? Even so, every good tree bears good fruit, but a bad tree bears bad fruit.* Because the seed that was sown was the Word of God, the people represented by the good ground will produce fruit generally conforming to the Word of God (both the written Scripture and the Living Word, Jesus Christ), although we recognize that we all are imperfect.

One form of fruit is honest thanksgiving, as described in Hebrews 13:15, which states, *Therefore by Him let us continually offer the sacrifice of praise to God, that is, the fruit of our lips, giving thanks to His name.* The ideal is thanksgiving from a thankful heart. Another is giving and sharing, as mentioned in 2 Corinthians 9:5-11. In that particular context, the generosity of the Corinthian church was to cause the Apostle Paul to give thanks to God. Paul also gave rejoiced for the generosity of the Philippian church, which supported Paul despite the poverty of its members. Philippians 4:10-20.

The most frequent usage of "fruit" in the New Testament relates to the new character being created in the maturing Christian. Consider the statement of Galatians 5:22-25:

> *But the fruit of the Spirit is love, joy, peace, longsuffering, kindness, goodness, faithfulness, gentleness, self-control. Against such there is no law. And those who are Christ's have crucified the flesh with its passions and desires. If we live in the Spirit, let us also walk in the Spirit.*

(There is also just prior to these verses a list of bad fruit that is to be purged because as converts we are not longer bad trees. Galatians 5:19-21; also compare Romans 1:18-32; 1 Corinthians 6:9-10, Colossians 3:5-10 and Revelation 9:20-21 for other summaries of evil fruit that should no longer exist in the life of a Christian and certainly should not characterize his or her new life. Consider also that in real-life "good ground" there are probably patches of thorns and areas of rock that need to be removed so that the whole area will bear fruit. So in some cases weeds are being removed almost simultaneously with good crops being planted. Love is listed first here because of its surpassing importance, as also expressed in 1 Corinthians 13:13 which reads, *And now abide faith, hope, love, these three; but the greatest of these is love.*

Colossians 3:12-17 is still another description of the fruit of Christianity which emphasizes the importance of love (possibly but not necessarily marital love, but love that puts other first as Christ Jesus put us first when He gave His life on the Cross for us):

> *Therefore, as the elect of God, holy and beloved, put on tender mercies, kindness, humility, meekness, longsuffering; bearing with one another, and forgiving one another, if anyone has a complaint against another; even as Christ forgave you, so you also must do. But above all these things put on love, which is the bond of perfection. And let the peace of God rule in your hearts, to which also you were called in one body; and be thankful. Let the word of Christ dwell in you richly in all wisdom, teaching and admonishing one another in psalms and hymns and spiritual songs, singing with grace in your hearts to the Lord. And whatever you do in word or deed, do all in the name of the Lord Jesus, giving thanks to God the Father through Him.*

While this passage does not use the word "fruit", it is so close in content to Galatians 5:22-25 that these should also be considered fruit of Christian character. When we are told to "put on" these things, the Holy Spirit through Paul is reminding us of our growing responsibility as a person who is growing out of spiritual infancy and even spiritual childhood toward maturity. As with natural children in physical families, God expects us to take more co-responsibility (never outside of the realm of the Spirit) as we mature.

2 Peter 1:5-8 is another list of Christian graces, but these are laid out in foundational sequence rather than in order of importance. Faith here is the first of the series because there is no Christian grace or virtue without faith first. If we try to manufacture other aspects of Christian character without saving faith, the whole structure will fail under stress. As the Holy Spirit states through Paul in Ephesians 2:8-9, *For by grace have you been saved through faith, and that not of yourselves. It is the gift of God, not of works, lest any man should boast.* The word "virtue" in 2 Peter 1:5-8 has a connotation of courage. Then consider the passage:

> *But also for this very reason, giving all diligence, add to your faith virtue, to virtue knowledge, to knowledge self-control, to self-control perseverance, to perseverance godliness, to godliness brotherly kindness, and to brotherly kindness love. For if these things are yours and abound, you will be neither barren nor unfruitful in the knowledge of our Lord Jesus Christ.*

For the purposes of the subject of this book, it is most important to note that "perseverance" is one of the necessary attributes of the Christian. We are to give all diligence to add to whatever perseverance we have. We also need to take care that our perseverance is directed to objectives that first of all comport with the Bible's teachings and then are part of God's plan for our individual lives. This will require at a minimum a life of regular Bible study, prayer and where possible a connection with a local church that prizes Christian truth and Christian character.

CHAPTER 4

DOES OUR ENDURANCE DEPEND ULTIMATELY ON US OR ON GOD?

Are you concerned about your ability to hold on to your faith? Do you remember the poster of the cat swinging on the end of a rope with the caption "Hang in there, baby"? Do you feel as if you are dangling at the end of your rope like the cat? Perhaps you remember the picture of the seagull starting to swallow the frog while the frog is starting to strangle the seagull. Maybe you feel like the frog or the seagull. If you truly depend on your own strength, your fears would make sense. So let's explore the Scriptures to see if your endurance in the final analysis depends on your strength or on God's everlasting love.

A good starting point is Romans 8:24-27, which reads:

> *For we were saved in this hope, but hope that is seen is not hope; for why does one still hope for what he sees? But if we hope for what we do not see, we eagerly wait for it with perseverance. Likewise the Spirit also helps in our weaknesses. For we do not know what we should pray for as we ought, but the Spirit Himself makes intercession for us with groanings which cannot be uttered. Now He who searches the hearts knows what the mind of the Spirit is, because He makes intercession for the saints according to the will of God.*

We are described as waiting with perseverance with the help of the Holy Spirit who prays for us. Can we truly imagine that the Spirit's intercession to the Father will not be heard favorably? Beyond the Spirit's intercession, there is also the prayer of Jesus Christ on our behalf. *Who is he who condemns? It is Christ who died, and furthermore is also risen, who is even at the right hand of God, who also makes intercession for us.* Romans 8:34. Can His prayer fail? Never! It was sufficient to preserve Peter from Satan (Luke 22:31-32), and His prayers will preserve us too. The Son of God and the Holy Spirit will never let go of us even if we lose our grip.

Example 1: The Apostle Paul

Let us examine whether the Apostle Paul's life was formed from his choices or from God's plan. If one thinks chronologically, one would start with Paul's birth. He first was known as Saul of Tarsus, but I will use the name under which he is famous for clarity. So far as we know, Paul's birth was ordinary in the physical sense, although we know that Paul was born a citizen of Rome instead of being merely a subject. This played a part in Paul's later ministry at least twice. (Acts 16:16-40, Acts 22:22-29) Another invisible but striking feature of Paul's birth is that he was already under the call of God, although Paul was a long way from understanding it. In Galatians 1:15-16 Paul writes that *"But when it pleased God, who separated me from my mother's womb and called me through His grace, to reveal His Son in me, that I might preach Him among the Gentiles, I did not immediately confer with flesh and blood ..."* So Paul was "separated from his mother's womb" even though he grew up to be an enemy of the Gospel and of the Church during his very young manhood, as is shown by his part in the stoning of the deacon Stephen in Acts 6-8. God permitted Paul's choices of his own original will to express themselves so long as they were consistent with His plan.

Then Paul headed away from Jerusalem for Damascus, as related in Acts 9. Paul's design was to arrest Christians there and drag them back to Jerusalem for trial. Because God was planning to send Paul away from Jerusalem, he allowed Paul to start on his plan. But then the risen Lord Jesus confronted and arrested Paul outside Damascus. When the Christian Ananias was commanded to go and baptize Paul, Ananias was shocked. Acts 9:10-14 can be summarized by an idea in Ananias' mind that God was either joking with him or testing him. But God was totally serious, as Acts 9:15-16 shows: *"But the Lord said to him [Ananias], 'Go, for he is a chosen vessel of Mine to bear My name before Gentiles, kings, and the children of Israel. For I will show him how many things he must suffer for My name's sake.'"* God has His own plan in operation, as shown by the word "chosen" in Acts 9:15. This dovetails with Paul's own testimony in Galatians 1 that he was separated from his mother's womb for the work. As further evidence of God's design in Paul's salvation, notice that Paul was the bear the name of Jesus Christ "before Gentiles, kings and the children of Israel." The order is precise and matches the course of Paul's later life during which his predominant witness was to Gentiles. His boyhood in Tarsus rather than in Israel was good training for Paul's later mission. Then Paul witnessed to Roman officials such as Sergius Paulus (Acts 13:6-12), Felix (Acts 24), Festus (Acts 25) and Agrippa (Acts 26). After these things Paul had hearings in Rome itself, which should have included the Emperor Nero although this is not recorded in Scripture. Paul witnessed to Jewish audiences also, especially among those scattered away from Jerusalem and Judea. But this was secondary to his witness to the Gentile world, in contrast to Peter. Galatians 2:7-8. Paul was told near the beginning of his ministry that those in Jerusalem would not listen to him (Acts 22:18-21, an excerpt of Paul's interrupted defense before the mob in Jerusalem when he was taken prisoner there). So it proved to be true.

God told the Ananias who baptized Paul that He would show Paul how many things Paul would suffer for Jesus' sake, before any of them had happened. Paul later summarized his physical sufferings in 2 Corinthians 11:23-33:

> *Are they ministers of Christ?-I speak as a fool-I am more: in labors more abundant, in stripes above measure, in prisons more frequently, in deaths often. From the Jews five times I received forty stripes minus one. Three times I was beaten with rods; once I was stoned; three times I was shipwrecked; a night and a day I have been in the deep; in journeys often, in perils of waters, in*

perils of robbers, in perils of my own countrymen, in perils of the Gentiles, in perils in the city, in perils in the wilderness, in perils in the sea, in perils among false brethren; in weariness and toil, in sleeplessness often, in hunger and thirst, in fastings often, in cold and nakedness; besides the other things, what comes upon me daily: my deep concern for all the churches. Who is weak, and I am not weak? Who is made to stumble, and I do not burn with indignation? If I must boast, I will boast in the things which concern my infirmity. The God and Father of our Lord Jesus Christ, who is blessed forever, knows that I am not lying. In Damascus the governor, under Aretas the king, was guarding the city of the Damascenes with a garrison, desiring to arrest me; but I was let down in a basket through a window in the wall, and escaped from his hands.

Up to the time of this epistle, which was written before Paul's imprisonments, Paul had had some hard traveling and would face more yet. I do not know precisely how many miles Paul walked on land during his missionary travels, but the number must be enormous. Yet again he would face the Mediterranean Sea (Acts 27) and snakebite (Acts 28:3-9). Given that Satan initially assumed the form of a snake, it is reasonable to regard the attack of the viper as symbolic of the attacks by Satan against Paul in efforts to bring Paul's ministry to a premature end. After this, imprisonment and martyrdom would follow. God knew about this suffering before it would happen, but Paul had to learn as he lived. But there can be no doubt that God had a detailed plan for Paul before Paul was ever converted to worship Jesus Christ. Neither can anyone doubt Paul's endurance through God's strength.

Example 2: Lord Jesus Christ

For a second example of God's pre-planning, consider a portion of the prophecies about the life of the Lord Jesus Christ. The following table references briefly a small portion of the prophecies that predate Jesus' birth by 400 years or more that were fulfilled in His life:

His birth in Bethlehem	Micah 5:2
Slaughter of babies by Herod	Jeremiah 31:15, quoted in Matthew 2:17-18
His coming out of Egypt	Matthew 2:15, quoting Hosea 11:1
His descent from David	2 Samuel 7:16, Matthew 1:6, Luke 3:31
Virgin Birth	Isaiah 7:14, Luke 1:27-35
Never a broken bone	Numbers 9:12, Psalm 34:19-20, John 19:32-36
Healed many	Isaiah 53:4, quoted in Matthew 8:17
Preach the gospel	Isaiah 61:1, Luke 7:20-22
Betrayal by close friend	Psalm 41:9; John 13:2,21-30
Rejection by majority	Psalm 69, Isaiah 53:3, John 1:10-11
Crucifixion and nakedness	Psalm 22, specially 22:16-17
Clothing parceled by lot	Psalm 22:18; John 19:24
Extreme thirst when dying	Psalm 22:14-15, Psalm 69:3, John 19:28
Rich man's grave	Isaiah 53:9, John 19:38-42
483 years from reconstruction of Jerusalem	Daniel 9:25-26
Raised from the dead on 3rd day	Psalm 16:10, quoted in Acts 2:27

The study of prophecy of Jesus Christ would take an entire lifetime and would justify many books. This brief selection is sufficient to show that God was working to a pre-determined plan in sending His Son Jesus Christ to the earth and receiving Him back into Heaven after His death, burial and resurrection. While God's plan for any of us is not of the same proportion as His plan for His Son Jesus Christ, He does have a definite plan for every one of His true children. As He followed through with Paul and with Jesus Christ, He will follow through with you and me.

Obstacles to God's plans

The Scriptures are clear that God's plans will not be frustrated but will be carried through to completion, as they were in the sacrificial death of Jesus Christ as a ransom for many as stated in Matthew 20:28. It is quite true that Satan tries to throw monkey wrenches into God's plans and in particular into His good plans for His people. 1 Peter 5:8-9 warns us to *"Be sober, be vigilant; because your adversary the devil walks about like a roaring lion, seeking whom he may devour. Resist him, steadfast in the faith, knowing that the same sufferings are experienced by your brotherhood in the world."* As we mature spiritually through godly training, we are sent into spiritual combat. But we are not alone. Peter earlier in the same letter (1 Peter 1:5) had told the believers that they are *"kept by the power of God through faith for salvation ready to be revealed in the last time."* The word "kept" literally means "guarded" or "garrisoned." Since we are "kept by the power of God" and because we know that Jesus Christ has already breached the Kingdom of Darkness through the Cross and the Resurrection (for example, see Hebrews 2:14, although this subject will receive greater discussion in Appendix A to keep to our main subject of endurance), we need not and should not fear the power of Satan, even though we are aware of its temporary existence within limits. With God's spiritual supply line to us secure, we can and will endure in the end through His power that keeps us.

Other Scriptures reinforce this lesson. Consider Jude 24-25, often quoted at the end of a church service. *"Now to Him who is able to keep you from stumbling* (the King James translation of *"falling"* will sound more familiar), *and to present you faultless before the presence of His glory with exceeding joy; to God our Savior, Who alone is wise, be glory and majesty, dominion and power, both now and forever. Amen."* The language "who is able" reminds one of Romans 14:4 in the context of a weak brother, *"Who are you to judge another's servant? To his own master he stands or falls. Indeed, he will be made to stand, for God is able to make him stand."* The weak servant stands because of the power of God, Who is able to make him stand. So in Jude the fact that God is able to keep us from falling implies a promise that He will do just that. Consider that in Hebrews 11:34 the heroes and heroines of faith *"out of weakness were made strong."* At the end of the day God's power will pull us through despite our weaknesses. We may be tempted to quit from spiritual or physical exhaustion, but He will supply and make good our lack of endurance to fulfill His promises.

We have already seen that God chose to send His Son into the world to save sinners and that He chose Paul no later than birth as His initially most visible apostle to the Greek and Latin world of the Roman Empire. God's choice extends to "ordinary" believers as well. A study of Romans 9-11 will confirm this. Furthermore, the Holy Spirit through Paul in Ephesians 1:3-5,7, 11 wrote that:

> *Blessed be the God and Father of our Lord Jesus Christ, who has blessed us with every spiritual blessing in the heavenly places in Christ, just as He chose us in Him before the foundation of the world, that we should be holy and without blame before Him, in love having predestined us to adoption as sons by Jesus Christ to Himself, according to the good pleasure of His will,*
>
> *In Him we have redemption through His blood, the forgiveness of sins, according to the riches of His grace*
>
> *In Him also we have obtained an inheritance, being predestined according to the purpose of Him who works all things according to the counsel of His will*

So we were actually chosen in Him before the foundation of the world, which probably means that we were chosen before God created time in Genesis 1:4-5. He also predestined us to the adoption as sons of God. He now have our redemption through His blood – we are not kept waiting to see how our lives turn out. We have already obtained an inheritance and have the Holy Spirit as a down-payment of the inheritance to come. (Ephesians 1:13-14) These facts indicate that God is working out His plan and will see us through as part of His grand design.

John 15:16 confirms the teaching that Jesus chose the disciples and not the other way around. *"You did not choose Me, but I chose you and appointed you that you should go and bear fruit, and that your fruit should remain, that whatever you ask the Father in My name He may give you."* So our fruit is in the last analysis ordained by God. As we mature in faith and grace, we will take more co-responsibility for our fruitfulness as for our endurance, but the overall power and direction remains with God as it has been from the beginning.

> *For by grace you have been saved through faith, and that not of yourselves. It is the gift of God, not of works, lest any man should boast. For we are His workmanship, created in Christ Jesus unto good works, which God has before ordained that we should walk in them. Ephesians 2:8-10.*

Objections to the idea of divine control

We know that the AntiChrist yet to come will cast deception such as has not been seen since Satan spoke through the snake in the Garden of Eden. Our Lord Jesus said that *"false christs and false prophets will rise and show great signs and wonders to deceive, if possible, even the elect."* Matthew 24:24 How will an "ordinary" believer see through a master deceiver like Satan when Eve was fooled (1 Timothy 2:14) before she had sinned, and Adam chose to follow her for his first sin even though he was not similarly deceived? Paul repeats the warning about false apostles in 2 Corinthians 11:13-15.

The first hint that it is not ultimately possible for the deception of the Devil to succeed ultimately in suborning the elect is the phrase "if possible" in Matthew 24:24. Our Lord Jesus commended the Ephesian church because they had *"tested those who say they are apostles and are not, and have found them liars."* Revelation 2:2. This does not mean that a believer may not be temporarily influenced by Satan as Peter was (Matthew 16:21-23), but rather that the believer will hold to the faith of Christ at the finish. Paul had confidence concerning the Philippian church that *"He who has begun a good work in you will complete it until the day of Jesus Christ."* Philippians 1:6.

In considering honest objections, there are three warning passages in Hebrews that some have interpreted as meaning that a true believer can lose his or her salvation – that he or she may not endure and that this is left up to each fallible human being. Since these passages are all in one letter, we should consider the context of that letter. Hebrews was written originally to Jews who had professed to believe that Jesus is Messiah, although it should be remembered that some in the congregations reading the letter may have been wavering under pressure from friends, family or other important people in their lives. Some hearers may have lacked saving faith when they heard the letter even though they were attending a Christian worship meeting. To be a Christian in Judea meant abandoning the traditional synagogue (John 9:22), which was the worship form that many of the Jews had known from childhood. When Peter and John taught in the Temple they were quickly arrested. (Acts 4:1-3) Others may have been attracted to the love and enthusiam of the believers without understanding the full truth about the Lord Jesus or being prepared for the ostracism that they would face for His Name's sake. There may have been a few spies meeting with the church. Galatians 2:4. Even they would be potential targets for the Gospel. Hebrews was meant to show the superiority of the New Covenant to the Old Covenant given by Moses and to show that Jesus was King and Messiah over Israel and Gentile alike. It also stresses elements of spiritual continuity between the saving faith in the coming Messiah exhibited by men such as Moses and King David and the saving faith in the crucified and risen Messiah taught by the new Christian Church. In this context are the great passages of warning about false faith that does not follow through to influence our thoughts and actions.

The first of these passages is Hebrews 3:6-19. The warning note is sounded first in verse 6, which introduces, *"Christ as a Son over His own house, whose house we are if we hold fast the confidence and the rejoicing of the hope firm to the end."* We have already seen in the Parable of the Soils that endurance and fruit are necessary consequences of saving faith, so we should not be surprised at this language nor at similar language in verse 14. Then the passage quotes from Psalm 95 as a warning against falling short of a complete, committed faith. The historical example used is the adult generation that left Egypt with Moses and yet fell short of the Promised Land and died in the Wilderness. If you start reading in Exodus 12 and the following chapters and continue with Numbers, you will find a constant litany of complaints starting immediately after God had parted the waters for them miraculously and had destroyed the Egyptian army to save them. This was the generation that persuaded Aaron to build the Golden Calf, which was destroyed. Their disobedient lack of faith climaxed when they refused to invade the Promised Land despite the encouragement of Joshua and Caleb. The congregation as a whole exhibited not occasional but consistent disobedience up to and including the refusal to enter the Promised Land. Paul in 1 Corinthians 10:5 summarized this generation: *"But with most of them God was not well pleased, for their bodies were scattered in the wilderness."* The Holy Spirit was warning the hearers of the letter to the Hebrews to be unlike that generation, which escaped their initial slavery only to fall short of the Promised Land of faith. Compare 2 Peter 2:20-22, dealing with people who temporarily escaped their polluted way of life but fell short of true faith and consequently went back to their old bondage to evil habits. Also consider Matthew 12:43-45 and Luke 11:24-26.

The next passage is Hebrews 6:4-12. Since we have already viewed the Parable of the Soils, verses 7-8 should not surprise us. We have already seen that soil that produces thorns symbolizes unsaved people. The start of the passage may seem to be more of a problem at first glance. How can a person who has tasted the heavenly gift and the good Word of God and has partaken of the Holy Spirit not have been saved during that time? Consider the case of Judas. He participated in the healing miracles of Matthew 10 and Luke 10. He was present at the other miracles of Jesus Christ. Judas had daily fellowship with Jesus. He appeared to the other disciples to be saved, so that none of them knew that Judas would be a traitor until Judas came to Gethsamane. (John 13:13-30) Another similar case seems to be Demas, who at first served with Paul but then loved this present world and deserted. (Philemon 24; Colossians 4:14; 2 Timothy 4:10). In the Old Testament King Saul and Ahithophel (David's counselor who deserted to Absalom – see 2 Samuel 15-17 for the complete story) are probably similar. All four of these were gifted and appeared faithful to God at first, but collapsed at the finish (unless Demas recovered and repented, which is not recorded in Scripture). In terms of Hebrews 6, I believe that these people tasted but spat out the good gifts of God for their own reasons, most likely because they may have wanted power on their own or preferred the wealth of this world to wealth in heaven. In that case Demas and those like him violate Matthew 6:19-33 and Hebrews 11:25-26 to their own destruction.

The most important point in the passage is verse 9, which says, *"But, beloved, we are confident of better things concerning you, yes, things that accompany salvation, though we speak in this manner."* The author was convinced of his readers' salvation even though he warned them from the examples of counterfeit believers in the past. The author was concerned lest there may be any unconverted people in the midst of the congregations but nothing shows that a genuinely saved person ever lost his or her salvation. The point of Hebrews 6 is to encourage the endurance that will sustain true hope all the way to the finish line, as stated in verse 11. Consider the passage as a whole as well as each of the individual parts.

The third great warning passage is Hebrews 10:26-39, which starts, *"For if we sin willfully after we have received the knowledge of the truth, there no longer remains a sacrifice for sins, but a certain fearful expectation of judgment, and fiery indignation which will devour the adversaries."* If we were to isolate these words from their context, we might think that to reach heaven we who believe must avoid any wilful sin whatsoever or face irretrievable ruin. I am not excusing sin in any form, but that isolated interpretation runs contrary to the rest of Scripture. For one example, the Apostle Peter withdrew from fellowship with Gentiles when he knew better (Galatians 2:11-19). How could the man who engaged in a sexual liaison with his father's wife (1 Corinthians 5:1-8 – note the hope for the man in v. 5) be forgiven and returned to the fellowship as commanded in 2 Corinthians 2:1-11 if one wilful sin after genuine salvation condemns a person to eternal fire? If one holds to such a theology, what can one say about King David, who certainly sinned wilfully concerning Uriah and Bathsheba after initial saving faith as evidenced by his victory over Goliath and especially David's Covenant with God as expressed in 2 Samuel 7? The idea that any wilful sin after saving faith triggers eternal damnation would expunge Psalms 32, 38 and 51 from the Scripture and also undermine the Roman epistle which draws heavily on Psalm 32 in Romans 4. Even Abraham lied to Abimelech about his marriage to Sarah after God had entered into covenant with him (Genesis 20:1-13 – the covenant is in

Genesis 15). Did John Mark, who later wrote the Gospel of Mark, sin wilfully by leaving Paul and Barnabas? (Acts 15:35-40) Probably. Was he doomed forever? No! Not only did he write the Gospel of Mark, but Paul himself later found John Mark profitable. 2 Timothy 4:11. Assuming that there are not two different "Marks", the same Mark who deserted Paul and Barnabas is mentioned in Colossians 4:10, Philemon 24 and 1 Peter 5:13. Moreover, such an isolated interpretation of Hebrews 10:26-27 would contradict verses 38-39 in the same context. The writer expresses confidence that not only himself but "we" – including at least a majority of his audience – *"are not of those who draw back to perdition, but of those who believe to the saving of the soul."* The previous verse quotes Habakkuk 2:4, which Paul quoted in Romans. *"The just shall live by faith."* Here is the central issue in all of the warning passages in Hebrews, including this one. Saving faith is essential to salvation. Thus, the "knowledge" in Hebrews 10:26 should be understood as intellectual awareness of the essential truths of the Gospel: that Jesus Christ was in fact the Son of God and sent from heaven to save many, and that He died, was buried and rose again according to the Scriptures. It is possible for a person to know these things and yet draw back from embracing them with joy and finally discard them for more immediate pleasure (contrast Moses in Hebrews 11:24-26). As James points out concerning faith that is intellectual only, *"The demons believe and tremble."* James 2:19.

No wonder that the writer of Hebrews says that *"For you have need of endurance, so that after you have done the will of God, you may receive the promise."* Hebrews 10:36. The initial hearers had already suffered financially for their beliefs, and more trouble was yet to come. From history we know that what the Romans called the Jewish War was not far off. We suspect that James, the half-brother of Jesus, was still alive when Hebrews was first written because his death is not mentioned (*"You have not yet resisted to bloodshed, striving against sin."* Hebrews 12:4). But he was soon to be murdered for his faith at the instigation of the unbelieving Temple leadership. The Jewish Christians in Judea would soon have to flee for their lives with only the clothes on their back. Matthew 24:16-20. The wilful sin which endangers the very soul of anyone is unbelief, the opposite of faith. In the case of one who has been an apparent Christian (for example, one represented by the stony or thorny ground in Matthew 13), unbelief would be a "drawing back" which triggers the special anger and displeasure of God. This is how the warnings of Hebrews should be understood without watering down their severity.

For indeed *"It is a fearful thing to fall into the hands of the living God."* Hebrews 10:31. The pains of God's eternal vengeance should not be scoffed at. They involve perpetual, unrelenting assaults on all of the senses and both physical and psychological pain unimaginable on earth. People often concentrate so much on the aspects of burning (true enough, *"Our God is a consuming fire."* Hebrews 12:29) that other aspects of everlasting punishment are overlooked. Indeed it is possible for a person to be beyond any hope of salvation even though still alive and physically healthy. In my student days I witnessed to a fellow student who quite courteously told me about himself. He was then bisexual. This in itself is forgivable. Note that in 1 Corinthians 6:9-11 some of the Corinthian converts had previously lived a life of sin in sexual matters. But then he told me that he had once believed in Jesus Christ and then had cast off his faith. To seal his renunciation he had used his Bible as toilet paper. When I tried to pray for him I felt a sensation of a cold, clammy hand over my mouth. God was refusing to even listen to my attempts to pray for that man. I had to either shut my mouth or change the subject. So far as it is given to me or any man to have such knowledge, I believe that this particular man is beyond hope if indeed he is still alive. He is a living example of one who cast off his faith and has committed the blasphemy of the Holy Spirit (Matthew 12:31-32).

God does not excuse sin, although He forgives it. The chastening of David for his sin in lusting after and finally murdering for Bathsheba was severe enough. Part of that chastening included the death of four children and a temporary period of flight during a civil war triggered by his son Absolom. But faith that transforms the entire person is the central issue of salvation. Without such faith, there is no salvation but damnation forever. That is the core of Hebrews. In that context we are told that *"we have need of endurance."* Hebrews 10:36. In context, this should be understood to imply that we must have faith that will persist to trust Jesus Christ through anything that we may face in this life.

As a final comfort, savor slowly and carefully and embrace the triumphant promises of God to every genuine believer in Romans 8:25-39:

> *But if we hope for what we do not see, we eagerly wait for it with perseverance. Likewise the Spirit also helps in our weaknesses. For we do not know what we should pray for as we ought, but the Spirit Himself makes intercession for us with groanings which cannot be uttered. Now He who searches the hearts knows what the mind of the Spirit is, because He makes intercession for the saints according to the will of God.*
> *And we know that all things work together for good to those who love God, to those who are the called according to His purpose. For whom He foreknew, He also predestined to be conformed to the image of His Son, that He might be the firstborn among many brethren. Moreover whom He predestined, these He also called; whom He called, these He also justified; and whom He justified, these He also glorified.*
> *What then shall we say to these things?*
> *If God is for us, who can be against us?*
> *He who did not spare His own Son, but delivered Him up for us all, how shall He not with Him also freely give us all things?*
> *Who shall bring a charge against God's elect? It is God who justifies. Who is he who condemns? It is Christ who died, and furthermore is also risen, who is even at the right hand of God, who also makes intercession for us.*
> *Who shall separate us from the love of Christ? Shall tribulation, or distress, or persecution, or famine, or nakedness, or peril, or sword? As it is written: "For Your sake we are killed all day long; We are accounted as sheep for the slaughter." Yet in all these things we are more than conquerors through Him who loved us.*
> *For I am persuaded that neither death nor life, nor angels nor principalities nor powers, nor things present nor things to come, nor height nor depth, nor any other created thing, shall be able to separate us from the love of God which is in Christ Jesus our Lord.*

CHAPTER 5

JOB: AN EXAMPLE OF ENDURING FAITH

The ordeal of Job was unusually severe but is still an example for us. James (5:10-11) exhorts us all to *"take the prophets, who spoke in the name of the Lord, as an example of suffering and patience. Indeed we count them blessed who endure. You have heard of the perseverance of Job and seen the end intended by the Lord-that the Lord is very compassionate and merciful."* Just before his ordeal, Job was a tremendously wealthy man with a wife and 10 healthy adult children. He had numerous transport animals, farm animals and broodmares. Job also had numerous employees who tended to the details of these business enterprises. His health was robust. With all this, Job worshipped God faithfully. In economic terms, he could be said to have been the Warren Buffett of his era, but also devout as were J.C. Penney and Willam Colgate.

Within an incredibly short time, all this was swept away in a series of cascading disasters orchestrated by Satan with God's permission. In modern terms, Job and his wife had 10 funerals in addition to tremendous property losses. From the Bible's description, a tornado killed the children. Job's property losses were not covered by insurance – even modern insurance excludes acts of war of the kind that seized Job's animals – and such insurance was probably not available to Job. In one day Job went from great wealth to almost nothing, and yet Job did not complain about his losses or accuse God of doing him wrong. Job 1:22.

When Satan could not induce Job to curse God with all this, Satan requested and received permission to attack Job's health. God gave permission with the limitation that Job could not be killed. Job was infected with boils, possibly the kind of boils that plagued the Egyptians before the Exodus. Boils of some type will again be part of the plagues of Revelation (16:2). Boils indicate infection, probable fever and great pain. In modern terms, imagine boils or bedsores caused by antibiotic-resistant bacteria. Job could not even stand up or lie down without pressing on some of his boils. This was enough to temporarily break the faith of Job's wife (Job 2:9) but Job never did "curse God and die." God seems to have passed over the sin of Job's wife in consideration of the terrible trial that she went through beside her husband. It is important that Job's wife never did leave him. God used her to rebuild the family after the ordeal.

Job still was a sinner and questioned God, but he never did curse Him or renounce his allegiance to and faith in God. Satan never did achieve his objective to induce Job to curse God. In this sense the patience of Job was a foreshadowing of Satan's defeat at every attempt to tempt the Lord Jesus (Matthew 4; Luke 4, Matthew 16:21-23 are the main instances).

Job wanted to present his case to God that he had not committed a heinous sin to provoke God to such apparent anger. In terms of Job's godliness compared to his fellow man, Job was correct, but Job was minimizing the most important point. Even the best of sinners fall so far short of the glory of God that they deserve nothing but His perpetual wrath and punishment. Only mercy can save them. Surely Job felt foolish when he could not answer even one of God's questions concerning His Creation starting in Job 38. Job grasped the truth that God was giving him, saying in Job 42:1-6:

> *Then Job answered the Lord and said: "I know that You can do everything, and that no purpose of Yours can be withheld from You. You asked, 'Who is this who hides counsel without knowledge?' Therefore I have uttered what I did not understand, things too wonderful for me, which I did not know.*
> *Listen, please, and let me speak; You said, 'I will question you, and you shall answer Me.'*

> "I have heard of You by the hearing of the ear, But now my eye sees You. Therefore I abhor myself, and repent in dust and ashes."

Job's friends who tried to comfort and counsel him did not "get it" as Job did. So Job offered sacrifices on their behalf as he had previously done for his children.

So this is the patience and spiritual endurance that James holds up as an example for us. While we may never have as much to lose as Job did, we know that the storms will blow on our life in a manner somewhat similar to the storms that overtook Job. (Matthew 7:24-27) Bearing in mind the awful condition of Job's body when he spoke each of these words, consider carefully the three towering expressions of faith that Job uttered in the midst of his agony:

> *Though He slay me, yet will I trust Him. Even so, I will defend my own ways before Him. He also shall be my salvation, for a hypocrite could not come before Him. Job 13:15-16*

> "For there is hope for a tree, if it is cut down, that it will sprout again, and that its tender shoots will not cease. Though its root may grow old in the earth, and its stump may die in the ground, yet at the scent of water it will bud and bring forth branches like a plant. But man dies and is laid away; indeed he breathes his last and where is he? As water disappears from the sea, and a river becomes parched and dries up, so man lies down and does not rise. Till the heavens are no more, they will not awake nor be roused from their sleep."

> "Oh, that You would hide me in the grave, That You would conceal me until Your wrath is past, That You would appoint me a set time, and remember me! If a man dies, shall he live again? All the days of my hard service I will wait, till my change comes. You shall call, and I will answer You; You shall desire the work of Your hands."

> For now You number my steps, but do not watch over my sin. My transgression is sealed up in a bag, and You cover my iniquity. "But as a mountain falls and crumbles away, and as a rock is

> *moved from its place; as water wears away stones, and as torrents wash away the soil of the earth; so You destroy the hope of man. You prevail forever against him, and he passes on; You change his countenance and send him away. Job 14:7-20*

Note the basics of Job's faith. He knows that his own iniquity is sealed up in a bag and has been separated from him. He also know that the best hopes and works of human beings are eroded, but Job does have the hope of the resurrection from the dead. In this next section Job emphasizes his sure hope of resurrection and also shows some early understanding of what was then the future redeeming sacrifice to come. Job first refers to his escape *"by the skin of my teeth"* (Job 19:20) and to the fact that even his wife and friends appear to be against him. But then Job turns from complaint to faith and says:

> *Oh, that my words were written! Oh, that they were inscribed in a book! That they were engraved on a rock with an iron pen and lead, forever! For I know that my Redeemer lives, and He shall stand at last on the earth. And after my skin is destroyed, this I know: That in my flesh I shall see God, Whom I shall see for myself, And my eyes shall behold, and not another. How my heart yearns within me! Job 19:23-27*

Such faith in the midst of such earthly misery astounded Satan and shocks the modern world. There is an old hymn "Give Me That Old-Time Religion" that expresses truth applicable to the patience of Job. That hymn points to Paul and Silas (probably thinking of their being jailed in stocks in Philippi – Acts 16:20-40) and also to Daniel, probably thinking of the lions' den. "It was good for Paul and Silas [in another verse, the prophet Daniel] and it's good enough for me." We should react the same way to Job's enduring faith passing all the way through terrible suffering and the blessing that followed. This faith was that (1) God had separated Job's sins from him; (2) That God would redeem (for us, has redeemed) him through a Redeemer, Whom we now know is Jesus Christ, His Son; and (3) We shall be resurrected from the dead (assuming that we die and are not raptured instead) and see God for ourselves in person. This faith sustained Job through his spiritual tunnel. I would add a verse to the old hymn:

> It was good for Job in grief;
> It was good for Job in loss;
> It was good for Job against Satan
> And it's good enough for me!

It should be good enough for us, even if we should be the generation that endures the termination of civilization as we now know it.

CHAPTER 6

JACOB: AN EXAMPLE OF ENDURANCE IN LIFE

Much of the second half of Genesis centers around Jacob. Although mild-mannered, he was hard-driving and unwilling to accept second place from the beginning of his life. Jacob struggled with Esau even in the womb. Genesis 25:23-24. When Esau came from the womb first, Jacob came after him grasping his heel. Genesis 25:26. Jacob lost no time in bargaining for Esau's birthright when he had a temporary advantage when the twins were older. Genesis 25:29-34.

This trait of ambition would make Jacob a difficult neighbor and a formidable competitor. Applied selfishly, ambition can create pride and deaden the soul. But ambition can be a motivating force for learning and improvement if directed properly. At first Jacob had a no-holds-barred approach to bettering himself at Esau's expense. His mother Rebekah concocted and Jacob executed a plan to divert the blessing that Isaac intended to give Esau to Jacob instead. The plan succeeded not because God approved the method but because the deception's success would fulfill the word that God had given to Rebekah before the twins were born. Consider Genesis 27 in the light of Genesis 25:23. Isaac was preparing to bless Esau contrary to the plan of God. While Rebekah's and Jacob's deceptive plan succeeded, there was a heavy price to pay. Jacob had to flee for his life and never saw his beloved mother again. Rebekah paid the corresponding price of having only Esau and his annoying wives (Genesis

26:34-35, 27:46) as companions in addition to her husband Isaac. Her beloved son was gone, not to be seen by her again as long as she lived on the earth.

So Jacob was on the run when God visited him in a dream at Bethel. He was not an attractive character. But we see no sign of self-pity in Jacob. He presses on to his uncle Laban and meets Rachel, his lifelong true love. He agreed to wait seven years for her and work for his uncle in the meantime. Yet the seven years flew by for Jacob and his wedding day arrived.

Although the Scriptures do not say so, from our knowledge of wedding celebrations we can reasonably infer that Jacob let his guard down during the wedding feast and perhaps drank more alcohol than usual (see Genesis 29 & 30 for this part of the narrative). This probably contributed to the success of Laban's deception in substituting Leah for Rachel in Jacob's wedding tent. But from our perspective we can see two other reasons why God permitted Laban's trick to succeed: (1) God gave Jacob a dose of his own medicine in permitting Jacob to be deceived in a similar way that he deceived his own father Isaac; and (2) That Rachel was not sufficiently strong to bear enough children on which to found the twelve tribes of Israel. Leah in fact bore six of the twelve Patriarchs plus one daughter. Rachel died during childbirth of her second child, Benjamin.

The sojourn of Jacob that was supposed to last a few days in fact lasted 20 years. During that entire time Jacob worked outdoors and lived in tents, fighting off wild animals to bring domestic animals to maturity. By no means was Jacob perfect, but he was hard-working and showed perseverance in cattle farming. Laban's own children complained that Jacob was getting rich at their expense. Jacob was obedient when God instructed him to leave Laban. (Genesis 31:3) But all of this is preliminary to the great encounter about to change Jacob's very soul forever.

Jacob had still to face Esau, who in Jacob's mind may still have been angry over the family birthright and blessing. No doubt this created anxiety in Jacob's mind. But the night before Jacob was going to cross the Jabbok into territory where Esau may be found, Jacob found himself in an unexpected wrestling match. I believe that the Son of God took quasi-human form to wrestle with Jacob, although some scholars may have an alternate explanation. Jacob had shown many unattractive traits in his previous life, but on this night he wrestled until daybreak. Genesis 32:24-32. We should not overlook this.

In my youth I was a wrestler for 5 years and on one occasion was able to prevail in an overtime bout of 8 minutes in a tournament. That was my third match in less than 24 hours. I also at Cane Spree in college lost a cane wrestling match that lasted nearly 25 minutes, an unusually long match. Both my opponent and I were "dead" at the end of that one. But our endurance pales to practically nothing compared to Jacob. Even if we think that the wrestling started about midnight, that meant a non-stop struggle between Jacob and the Son of God of about 6 hours. This estimate is probably too short. But as a former wrestler I know that even 6 hours of non-stop wrestling is an extraordinary feat of physical endurance. If you doubt me, ask any wrestling coach how many 6-hour practices he has run without a break. About 3 to 3½ hours was the longest I remember, and those were rare. Even in these there were breaks for instruction and demonstration.

In this encounter with the Son of God, Jacob showed his cardinal virtue, his endurance and perseverance. This virtue is so important that God chose to identify Himself by Jacob's name: *"I am ... the God of Abraham, the God of Isaac and the God of Jacob."* Exodus 3:6. Ideally, we would pray with the vigor with which Jacob wrestled.

There were three main results that came from Jacob's wrestling with God. First, Jacob from then on sought the blessing of God as he had once sought the blessing of Isaac, his human father. Jacob knew that his Father in heaven was his true strength and source of blessing. Jacob would not let go without a blessing no matter how exhausted he was. Second, Jacob was thereafter disabled physically with a damaged hip so that he could no longer rely on his own strength but was forced to rely on God instead. Third, Jacob (=supplanter) was renamed Israel (=Prince with God) to match his newly transformed focus. In the main, Jacob's natural perseverance would be redirected from the pursuit of his own wealth and security to pursuing God and in trusting Him and receiving blessing from Him.

Jacob's later trials were more emotional and psychological than physical. He endured droughts. He was concerned about retaliation for Simeon's and Levi's treacherous attack on the men of Shechem. Rachel died in childbirth. Probably the worst anxiety was over Joseph, who had been supposedly killed but was actually sold into slavery by his half-brothers. Once again Jacob was on the receiving end of deception, this time by his own children. And once again God turned evil into good. (See Joseph's understanding in Genesis 50:20.)

Even at Jacob's worst, I cannot find a place in his life when he quit. On the very last day of his life he prophesied concerning his posterity (Genesis 49). If we are to pass through death instead of rapture, then let this Scripture be true of us:

> *Who can count the dust of Jacob, or number one-fourth of Israel?*
> *Let me die the death of the righteous, and let my end be like his!*
> Numbers 23:10

CHAPTER 7

ASPECTS OF MOSES' ENDURANCE

If one were to read Hebrews 11 – the great chapter of the faithful people of God – one would find many examples not only of faith but of endurance also. I will focus briefly on one more giant of faith, Moses. His life divides into thirds of forty years each. As a baby he escaped genocide through the providence of God orchestrating a combination of wise parents who complied literally with Pharaoh's law requiring that male children be thrown into the Nile River and a compassionate Egyptian princess who had the courage to stand up to her murderous father. Thus Moses grew up as an Egyptian prince and received a first-class education in Egyptian knowledge. When forty, he decided to visit his biological relatives and was horrified at what he saw, to the point of killing an Egyptian overseer in the defense of a fellow Hebrew. Then the next 40 years were years of exile and tending livestock as did Jacob. Moses married and had one son during this interval, but lived a hard, physical outdoor life that toughened his body. He also had plenty of time alone to think and meditate. At long last Moses encountered God in the burning bush when he was 80 years old and was sent back to Egypt to liberate Israel.

The final third of Moses' life was extraordinary and called for extraordinary endurance. Just recalling the highlights gives an idea of the tremendous endurance required. First came the confrontations with Pharaoh and the Ten Plagues. Then the Passover and the Feast of Unleavened Bread were instituted. The Exodus itself occurred, with the final escape of Israel from the Egyptian Army taking place when the

Egyptians were drowned as the waters of the Red Sea closed over its normal channel.

The destruction of the Egyptian army had momentous consequences for all of the politics of the Middle East which have never subsided completely. For most of the time between Abraham and Moses, Egypt was the predominant power in the land we now call Israel. After Moses and Joshua, this was never true again for any extended period of time despite periodic attempts by Egypt to reassert its control. The main attempts came after Solomon's death and again after the death of Josiah before Babylon became the first of four great empires (Babylon, Persia, Greece and Rome) to control the Holy Land. But all of Egypt's attempts to regain control of the Holy Land failed. Even in the 20th century, Egypt (now under Arab rule instead of the rule of the people of ancient Egypt) was unable in 1948, 1967 or 1973 to gain control of the Holy Land. Moses is truly an epochal figure in both military history and in law.

When reading Exodus (and then Numbers for historical sequence, with Leviticus being mostly the book of the priesthood), one might think that Moses' work was coming to an end after the destruction of the Egyptian army because the road to the Holy Land was now open without opposition by a major military power. But this did not turn out to be true. Israel needed to be organized. The worship of God had to be set in order. The Covenant, highlighted by the Ten Commandments on two stone tablets, needed to be taught to the people. But even after all of the miracles the older generations had seen, they lacked faith and tried Moses' patience and even angered God Himself. The people first started to complain that they were not receiving enough food and water. When God supplied those, the stubborn people complained about the lack of variety and wanted meat. God gave them so much quail that it came out of their ears. The people pressured Aaron into making an idol – the Golden Calf. Moses supernaturally endured 40 days without food or water when God made the second set of the Ten Commandments. Exodus 34:28. The people on several occasions accused Moses (and indirectly, God Himself) of leading them into the Wilderness to die there. Some of the Levites rebelled at the leadership of Moses and Aaron. Even Aaron's sister complained about Moses' second wife. The climax of the older generations' unfaithfulness was their refusal to follow Joshua's and Caleb's leadership to conquer the Holy Land which they had been promised. When this refusal was completed, God vowed to kill off the older generation little by little in favor of those who had been under 20 years old at the time of the Exodus.

I relate this very compressed history of the generation of the Exodus to highlight Moses' endurance during the final third of his life. (If you really want a thorough spiritual exposition of the history of Israel from the Exodus until Joshua attacked Jericho, try to find volumes by A.W. Pink on this subject. These are not the most recent but they will richly repay months or even years of study with an open Bible and an honest heart.) Moses more than once interceded for Israel when God had just cause to destroy them. (Exodus 32:7-14 and Numbers 14 are two major examples) Moses lost his temper only once, recorded in Numbers 20:1-13. For this reason he did not enter the Promised Land during his physical life, although he was brought by the Lord Jesus to the Mount of Transfiguration to be present with Peter, James and John, the inner core of the disciples. Through God Moses did have extraordinary physical stamina, as shown by the comment that he was still vigorous and even able to enjoy relations with his second wife right up to his death at age 120. (Deuteronomy 34:7) But this is secondary to Moses' ability to put up with a stubborn, rebellious nation with only a few with whom he could have real fellowship. This is the unique aspect of Moses' patience and endurance.

Perhaps you have a difficult person in your life. Joyce Landorf once wrote a book entitled <u>Irregular People</u>. If so, take heart. Moses dealt patiently and wisely with a whole generation opposed to God and maintained his faith and even his patience and endurance. The same God who sustained Moses through these trials can sustain you.

CHAPTER 8

ENDURANCE AFTER FALTERING – THE EXAMPLE OF ELIJAH

Elijah was the other man brought with Moses to the Mount of Transfiguration by our Lord Jesus. Elijah was the first full-time prophet to Israel, although he did not write so far as we know. We do know that he first told the wicked King Ahab of the coming drought. During the drought God miraculously sustained him first at the Brook Cherith and then at the home of a Gentile woman at Zarephath, just northwest of Israel. Elijah through the power of God raised her only son from the dead. In the meantime Israel had no rain for over 3 years, and Ahab was desperate. Elijah came back into Israel and met Obadiah, a godly servant of a most ungodly king. Elijah then challenged both Ahab and the prophets of Baal to a contest. Each side would set up a sacrificial altar with wood and a sacrificed animal. The prophets of Baal would call upon Baal; Elijah would call upon the God of Israel. *"The God Who answers by fire, He is God."* The entire religious history of the world hung in the balance, but Elijah was so sure of the truth that he had scarce and precious water to soak the altar and fill a trench so that the anticipated fire would not burn the people along with the sacrifice and the altar. We all know the rest of the story as told in 1 Kings 18. Baal did not answer; the God of Israel did answer by fire. Elijah was so physically charged that he was able to outrun Ahab's chariot back to the city. The priests of Baal were killed and the people professed faith in the God of

Israel. Ahab was displeased, but his wife Queen Jezebel was livid. She threatened Elijah's life.

At this point Elijah faltered instead of showing the resolution he had shown up to this point. He ran for his life all the way to Beersheba, which was in Judah and therefore beyond Ahab's and Jezebel's jurisdiction. As Richard Nixon was to write about 2750 years later in Six Crises before he became President, Elijah found the time of spiritual and physical exhaustion after the main confrontation to be the most dangerous part of his spiritual battle. As you read the account in 1 Kings 19, consider that God was not harsh on Elijah. First God let Elijah sleep. For some this is the most healing thing possible, even spiritually. Psalm 127:2. The angel that God sent twice gave Elijah food and water to sustain Elijah on his journey. Like Moses, Elijah supernaturally endured 40 days without food or water after the angel's provisions. Then God revealed Himself to Elijah not in the fury of judgment but in the still, small voice of peace. Finally, God gave Elijah three further instructions before He would take Elijah home to Himself. Elijah had to anoint Hazael King over Syria and have Jehu anointed in the place of Ahab as King of Israel. Elijah also had to anoint Elisha and to prepare Elisha to replace himself as prophet. So Elijah, discouraged as he had become, could see an end to his labor and drew renewed courage from the prospect of the finish line, much as a distance runner perks up when he or she can see the finish.

I am not trying to make any assessment of Richard Nixon as a man or as a President. However, his later life proves that his basic point in Six Crises was true. The most mentally and spiritually dangerous time for a man or woman is after the central battle has been fought, because it is so natural to let one's guard down. Richard Nixon's worst moments as President came during his second term, after he had won his final election campaign and when his greatest stress should have been over. President Nixon forgot his own lesson, but his original lesson was correct and serves as a good explanation of Elijah's reaction after God answered Elijah's prayer by fire.

Elijah, though exhausted spiritually and physically following the confrontation with the prophets of Baal, was still sufficiently wise to fall toward God and to seek Him rather than to fall away or run away

from God even as he faltered. If you are at the end of your strength and cannot go on, fall toward Him instead of away from Him. God is a merciful and gracious God. God not only empowered Elijah to go on to finish his service but also sent a chariot with angels to spare Elijah physical death. Like Enoch, He was raptured instead.

CHAPTER 9

SAMSON: ENDURANCE AFTER COLLAPSE

Is it possible to regain endurance after moral collapse? If one repents, then yes. So many illustrious people, even with earthly riches, have driven their own lives into a ditch. Tiger Woods is one of the most recent examples, but he is far from alone. Political leaders from both major parties have made shipwreck of their marriages, not to mention movie stars and music singers. A generation ago, Jim Bakker was in a similar position, and he has admitted how far he strayed in his book *I Was Wrong*. If you are tempted to stray sexually from faithful monogamous marriage (or from celibacy if unmarried), read the first 10 chapters of Proverbs and then the appropriate section of Jim Bakker's book as a reality check before you plunge off the deep end.

In the realm of finance, Michael Milken in the 1980s seemed to have it all. He was a pioneer in "junk bond" financing. However, he ran afoul of the securities laws and went to prison and was forever barred from the securities industry. When he was released, he became involved in attempts to research cancer cures. Milken today has regained a certain respect for his charitable efforts after his release. So far as I am aware, he has never said anything about faith. His illustration lacks the spiritual dimension of salvation coming from Chuck Colson, who went from hard-boiled White House counselor in the Nixon White House to prisoner to a great spiritual leader known especially for his ministry to prisoners, even around the world.

Chuck Colson has had one of the most dramatic spiritual transformations of the 20th century. But Michael Milken to my knowledge has not spoken of spiritual influences, and Chuck Colson's change came through a new faith in Christ that he did not have in the White House. Neither of these examples deal with the professing Christian who has strayed while professing his faith. One can refer to King David and Bathsheba. We have already mentioned Psalms 38, 51 and 32; David makes scattered references in other Psalms to his fall and spiritual restoration through the mercy of God. But Samson's story is tailor-made for the person who has had a major spiritual collapse and wonders whether he or she can ever be restored to fellowship with God. Samson's story is told in Judges 13-16.

If we want to start off with physical endurance, Samson had that in spades. He killed a thousand Philistine fighters with the jawbone of an ass. Judges 15:15. He was capable of lifting an entire city gate out of the city wall and carrying the gate up and down hills. Judges 16:3. If there had been a "World's Strongest Man" competition in Samson's time, it would not have been a contest at all. Samson would have won hands down.

For men especially, great strength and athletic ability and sexual temptation tend to go together. Part of this is physiological; testosterone is positively correlated with both athletic ability and sexual desire. Part is psychological; some women will fling themselves at athletes. Solomon warned, *"For by means of a harlot a man is reduced to a crust of bread; and an adulteress will prey upon his precious life."* Proverbs 6:26. Such diverse athletic figures as Wade Boggs, Magic Johnson, Wilt Chamberlain and Tiger Woods have found this to be true to their sorrow. Sexual temptation is not the only way a man or woman can go astray, but it is a repeated theme in Scripture and also in contemporary society. So the very abundance of testosterone that will help a man excel as an athlete is also a source of weakness in the direction of sexual temptation. Samson is certainly an illustration.

Samson's strength was not just testosterone. It was that he had been dedicated to the Lord God as a Nazirite and as a sign of that vow had not cut his hair. A Nazirite was to be pure. Samson for some reason was attracted to Philistine women even though his commission was to free Israel from Philistine domination. For the 20 years when Samson judged

Israel it seems that this lust was held in check, but it was not extinguished. It is unlikely that the Philistine women shared Samson's belief in God. The pattern is consistent from his initial marriage in Judges 14 through the prostitute in Gaza mentioned in Judges 16:1 to his *femme fatale* Delilah in Judges 16:4. Such an analogous spiritual mismatch is to be avoided by any Christian believer today. The consequences are likely to be disastrous as were the consequences of Samson's confession to Delilah about the source of his strength. Instead of protecting Samson's confidence, Delilah betrayed him for money. This is entirely to be expected from any person, male or female, who does not fear God and has not been transformed from the original birth nature by Jesus Christ. Samson wound up with his eyes gouged out and bound to a grinding wheel like an animal, being goaded and whipped to keep the grinding wheel turning. Life seemed hopeless at this point.

But no situation is hopeless if God is present. The Scriptures tell us that Samson's hair began to grow back (Judges 16:22). The Philistine elite decided to throw a party with Samson as a comedy act. He had killed so many Philistines – they were going to celebrate the "fact" that he was now permanently helpless. But God turned the joke on the Philistines. Samson was able to decoy his handlers into letting him lean against the main supports of the building. We find that Samson was able to pray again. *Then Samson called to the Lord, saying, "O Lord God, remember me, I pray! Strengthen me, I pray, just this once, O God, that I may with one blow take vengeance on the Philistines for my two eyes!"* Judges 16:28. Then Samson's final prayer was *"Let me die with the Philistines!"* Judges 16:30. God answered both prayers. Because of Samson's previous sin, he was in a situation where praying for death made sense. Nevertheless, he did begin to liberate Israel from the iron grip of the Philistines. Looking back on his entire life, the Holy Spirit classified Samson as a hero of faith (Hebrews 11:32). By all means we must learn the spiritual lessons from Samson's fall, which in his case was triggered by unlawful sexual lust that was not put to death (compare Romans 8:13 – *For if you live according to the flesh you will die; but if by the Spirit you put to death the deeds of the body, you will live.*). But we must equally learn from Samson's final recovery, that if we repent God is gracious to restore our ability to pray (compare Psalm 66:18:

If I regard iniquity in my heart, the Lord will not hear me.) and to resume His grace in the place where we find ourselves as a consequence of our sin. **Samson is another major example of the truth that God does not let go of us even when we let go of Him.**

CHAPTER 10

SNAPSHOTS OF ENDURANCE

Like the writer of Hebrews in chapter 11 in dealing with faith (Hebrews 11:32-33), I realize that I cannot cover all the examples of endurance in the Scriptures. I do not wish to make reading this book a marathon! I therefore will comment briefly about Noah, who build an Ark and warned his contemporaries for a period of 120 years with no results beyond his family. I can imagine that Noah's neighbors thought him crazy to build an ark when it had never rained on the earth. But Noah listened to God and built the Ark (really a barge or an enclosed raft) according to God's instructions. Noah had no previous experience as a shipwright. Through perseverance Noah finished on time, resulting in the salvation of his family and of samples of air-breathing life to replenish the earth after the Flood.

Daniel the prophet was born in or near Jerusalem in Jeremiah's time and witnessed the moral collapse of Jerusalem after King Josiah's death in battle. That moral collapse was mirred by military collapse with Babylonian forces under Prince Nebuchadnezzar taking the city. Daniel was one of the first wave of captives taken to Babylon, where he was promptly castrated and then put in a training school for Babylonian bureaucrats. This was a rough start. The castration in Temple terms made Daniel unfit for worship, but that never seems to have bothered him so far as the Scriptures inform us. This also accounts for the lack of any mention of Daniel's family. His captors had made that impossible before Daniel was old enough to think about it.

Daniel's first crisis after his castration and placement in training school was the issue of diet – apparently the Babylonians wanted Daniel to eat food forbidden by the Law of Moses. Through precocious diplomatic skill Daniel was able to keep his conscience clean and continue his training. His second crisis was the command by King Nebuchadnezzar that all of the wise men of Babylon should be killed because they could not tell the king both a secret dream and its interpretation. God revealed the dream and its interpretation to Daniel in a night vision so that the King was assuaged. Daniel's three friends were thrown into a furnace for refusing to worship an image of gold made at Nebuchadnezzar's direction, but they survived the fire. Then the pride of King Nebuchadnezzar (who had become Daniel's patron after he revealed the dream) caused his insanity and temporary downfall. Daniel was not so popular with Nebuchnezzar's successors because, unlike Nebuchadnezzar himself (see Daniel 4 for Nebuchnezzar's account of his final worship of the God of Israel), they did not learn the lesson of humility or of the sovereignty of God. So the next crisis came when King Belshazzar decided to drink wine using the articles plundered from the Jewish Temple. That night Daniel survived the downfall of the Babylonian Empire which had trained him and survived to take high office under the early Media-Persians. But his rivals in the government persuaded King Darius to outlaw prayer to anyone but the King for 30 days. Daniel prayed to God –law or no law– and promptly was thrown into the lions' den. Daniel survived that and saw the downfall of his enemies and lived to a ripe old age.

Daniel is probably the best Secretary of the Treasury anyone ever had. He was faithful and honest. His endurance in government service from a teenager to an old man through a complete regime change shows the hand of God on him. I suspect that Mordecai (the uncle of Queen Esther) was either trained by Daniel or trained by someone who had been trained by Daniel. Certainly physical strength played no part in Daniel's endurance as it did for the earlier part of Jacob's life – his early castration deprived him of that burst of testosterone that would have made him physically strong. Daniel was faithful from his diet as a youth to his prayer as an aged man. When King Belshazzar offered to honor Daniel, Daniel turned him down flat. Daniel's endurance was spiritual and mental. He was sufficiently pure in heart and soul that God entrusted to Daniel the tremendous relevations of the 4 empires and of the coming of Messiah during the 4th Empire – Rome.

King David's life is well worth a book by itself. When weighing his endurance for a quick sketch, there is hardly a time when his life was free from conflict once he was anointed King in Saul's place. David almost always seemed to have at least one enemy. Goliath, Saul, Ishbosheth (Saul's son and rival for the throne after Saul's death), Michal (Saul's daughter and David's first wife who opposed David's worship when bring the Ark to Jerusalem) Absolom and Adonijah are just a few, and none of these after Goliath were from the surrounding countries whom David fought for the sake of Israel's national security. Near the end of his life David had to intervene to install Solomon and block Adonijah from seizing the throne. Even David's army commander Joab was a problem. David's conduct with respect to Uriah and Bathsheba was terrible, but David never lost faith and endured trusting in God to the end. David endured!

To reinforce the point that physical strength is not essential to endurance, I would comment briefly on the contemporary life of Joni Erickson Tada, who was paralyzed in a terrible diving accident as a teenager. Her very condition excludes physical strength because she can control only her head and neck. Joni refused to shrivel into a shell after her terrible injury. She learned to compose art by holding a pencil or brush between her teeth and controlling her instrument with her neck. Then she has become an author. She is one of the most joyous well-known Christian women today. Her endurance of her challenges with joy should silence any one of us who are inclined to complain.

CHAPTER 11

JESUS CHRIST AS AN EXAMPLE OF ENDURANCE

Our ultimate example in endurance as in any other virtue is our Lord Jesus Christ. One can observe the initial physical aspects of His endurance in the walks he took around the Holy Land and in the areas bordering it. These were not unique. All of the disciples accompanied Him, and in total mileage Paul certainly surpassed Him because of the length and reach of Paul's ministry. While our Lord Jesus was in terrific physical condition, that was not the core of His endurance.

Our Lord Jesus had at least two broad missions: to actually pay in full for the sins of His people and to be our complete and supreme example of how to live and what kind of person to be. Physical endurance was secondary to spiritual and mental endurance for Him.

Consider that on at least one occasion He spent all night in prayer to God, skipping sleep completely. Luke 6:12. In my own experience prayer is some of the hardest work I do. I can identify with Peter and the other disciples at Gethsamane, who fell asleep while trying to pray and could not last one hour in prayer. Matthew 26:38-45; Mark 14:37-41; Luke 22:45. Jesus' prayer time with His Father on the occasion of praying through the night lasted 7 or 8 hours with no vain repetition nor any wandering of mind. Extraordinary! We know this because Jesus was Perfect Man as well as the Son of God. Except in an extreme crisis, I would not recommend trying this nor total sleep deprivation, but Jesus' ability to endure this is an indication of how far beyond us He truly is. His example should be a spur for most of us to expand our prayer time and ministry.

Another sample of Jesus' endurance is found in John 6. A parallel account is found in Matthew 14 following the news of the death of John the Baptist. Our Lord Jesus first healed many people and then fed 5000 men, plus their dependents, from 5 loaves and 2 fish. There were even leftovers. Following that our Lord Jesus went to a mountain to pray alone while the disciples were crossing the lake. In the small hours of the morning Jesus was walking across the lake and invited Peter to walk toward Him on the water. When the crowds caught up with the Lord Jesus the next day, He preached to them a message about Himself as the Bread of Life. Contemplate accomplishing this in 24 hours without motorized transport. The endurance, both physical and especially spiritual and mental, is inconceivable for us in our mortal bodies with limited minds with limited spiritual vision. Let this packed 24-hour period be a sample of the entire public ministry of our Lord Jesus.

Hebrews 5:8 teaches that Jesus Christ *"learned obedience by the things which He suffered."* If we concentrate of the last hours of Jesus' life, we will remember that while praying for the future church at Gethsemane that He sweat drops of blood even though Jesus was strengthened by an angel. Luke 22:43-45. Right after this Jesus submitted to arrest even though He could have called angels to fight on His behalf. Matthew 26:53. He endured two night-time trials, though trial at night was illegal. He endured a horrific beating roughly as portrayed in *The Passion of the Christ*, though the real thing was worse than the movie. He struggled to carry the crossbar of His cross through Jerusalem streets to Golgotha. He was spiked to the Cross and mocked by His judges. Even the robbers crucified with Him at first mocked Him. This was the climax of the human rejection that had been a consistent pattern during His life and persists even today. More than this, He endured the rejection of His Father Whom He had known for eternity because that rejection was part of the punishment for the sins of His people. No wonder Jesus on the Cross quoted Psalm 22:1: *My God, My God, why have You forsaken Me?* He endured extreme thirst and excruciating pain. He endured the darkness that fell during His time on the Cross. Through such things Jesus Christ, Who always had been equal to His Father, learned obedience as a subordinate. This section could be summarized by Philippians 2:5-13:

> *Let this mind be in you which was also in Christ Jesus, Who, being in the form of God, did not consider it robbery [I might paraphrase this "did not think it something to be clung to"] to be equal with God, but made Himself of no reputation, taking the form of a bondservant, and coming in the likeness of men. And being found in appearance as a man, He humbled Himself and became obedient to the point of death, even the death of the cross. Therefore God also has highly exalted Him and given Him the name which is above every name, that at the name of Jesus every knee should bow, of those in heaven, and of those on earth, and of those under the earth, and that every tongue should confess that Jesus Christ is Lord, to the glory of God the Father. Therefore, my beloved, as you have always obeyed, not as in my presence only, but now much more in my absence, work out your own salvation with fear and trembling; for it is God who works in you both to will and to do for His good pleasure.*

Our Lord Jesus also endured contact with Satan, including being tempted by him. See Matthew 4 and Luke 4 for this account. Since our Lord Jesus was and is perfectly holy and Satan is unalloyed evil, this confrontation must have been supremely uncomfortable. Likewise, Jesus endures us and other sinners even though He has the power to destroy immediately and totally. As Hebrews 12:3 says, *"For consider Him who endured such hostility from sinners against Himself, lest you become weary and discouraged in your souls."* When His disciples could not heal a child, Jesus said in Matthew 17:17-18: *"O faithless and perverse generation, how long shall I be with you? How long shall I bear with you? Bring him here to Me." And Jesus rebuked the demon, and it came out of him; and the child was cured from that very hour.* Romans 9:22-24 asks this question about God, which question applies equally to our Lord Jesus:

> *What if God, wanting to show His wrath and to make His power known, endured with much longsuffering the vessels of wrath prepared for destruction, and that He might make known the*

riches of His glory on the vessels of mercy, which He had prepared beforehand for glory, even us whom He called, not of the Jews only, but also of the Gentiles? [Other translations may use "fitted" in place of "prepared". My interlinear Greek-English New Testament uses "fitted" as a literal translation, stressing more the moral state of the vessels of destruction and less on the decree of God. Both ideas are in fact true and are shown in many Scriptures. For example, in Romans 9:17-18 Pharaoh was raised up so that God could throw him down. See also Jude 4 for a passage that stresses the decree of God concerning false teachers before they were born. It seems that this particular verse focuses primarily on the aspect that the vessels of destruction richly deserve to be destroyed.]

So our Lord Jesus exhibited great patience and endurance in His life on earth and shows the same character now. Yet so often we respond to Him by cursing His name and showing ingratitude even if we restrain our curses. How unworthy we are and how merciful He is! As we grow in faith, we need to learn and exhibit more of His patience and endurance. On the earth, Jesus held back His power to accomplish his missions of being a supreme example and of paying for our sins on the Cross. When He returns, He will unleash His power as is shown in both 1 and 2 Thessalonians and especially in Revelation.

CHAPTER 12

WHY DO WE NEED ENDURANCE?

A. To reap natural and spiritual fruit

In the natural world, any farmer knows that he needs patience and endurance. James used this natural truth as an illustration: *"Therefore be patient, brethren, until the coming of the Lord. See how the farmer waits for the precious fruit of the earth, waiting patiently for it until it receives the early and latter rain. You also be patient. Establish your hearts, for the coming of the Lord is at hand."* James 5:7-8. Farmers around that world know that there is a long interval between sowing and reaping. In between, the farmer has to trust God for normal water and sunshine. At the right time the farmer must apply fertilizer for an optimum crop. Many crops have natural enemies that have to be countered. For fruit pollinating agents are necessary. With the decline of European honeybees and the spread of aggressive Africanized bees, this cannot be taken for granted. In short, the perceptive farmer learns the need for faith, then endurance as he waits for harvest, and then further endurance to actually reap the harvest.

The Apostle Paul in Galatians 6:9 exhorts us, *"Let us not grow weary while doing good, for in due season we shall reap if we do not lose heart"* (King James *"if we faint not"*). For example, Paul stayed in Corinth 18 months, working and laboring to establish a Christian congregation. Acts 18:11. At the beginning Paul worked as a tentmaker to support himself while he was teaching in the Jewish synagogue on sabbath days. Acts 18:3-4.

Nor was Paul alone in establishing the Corinthian church. 1 Corinthians 3:5-6. While God was giving the increase, He was using human beings like ourselves – to be sure, human beings with special gifts from the Holy Spirit – to work the ground and sow the good seed of the Word, leading to the harvest. We do not have the precise instructions nor the same personal authority of the Apostle Paul, but we all share responsibility for the Great Commission. Matthew's version is recorded in Matthew 28:18-20:

> *Jesus came and spoke to them, saying, "All authority has been given to Me in heaven and on earth. Go therefore and make disciples of all the nations, baptizing them in the name of the Father and of the Son and of the Holy Spirit, teaching them to observe all things that I have commanded you; and lo, I am with you always, even to the end of the age." Amen.*

We are to be contributing to the fulfillment of the Great Commission in some fashion. We should expect that instant conversions will be rare and that our efforts to witness will provoke opposition. Our Lord Jesus was loved by some but He was also the most hated Man of His generation. About thirty years later it was Jesus' half-brother James who was so hated that he was tossed off the pinnicle of the Temple. Josephus, the historian, records this as the fuse that triggered the explosion of the Jewish War which ended in the destruction of the Temple, of Jerusalem and of all Israel. Paul provoked controversy in most places that he preached. For example, it was said in Thessalonica by enemies of the Gospel that *"These who have turned the world upside down have come here too."* Acts 17:6. In truth we are turning the world rightside up, but we cannot expect those who do not know the Lord Jesus as a living person to perceive that. Opposition in some form is par for the course for witnesses for Jesus Christ. Therefore we need endurance to face and overcome spiritual obstacles.

Corinth was not the only instance of Paul spending extended time to establish a Christian church. In Ephesus Paul spent two years. Acts 19:10. In Ephesus, note also the attempts by the seven sons of Sceva to counterfeit the miracles of Paul as one form of spiritual opposition. The silversmiths who were losing money because they were selling fewer idolatrous statuettes of Diana tried to organize a riot or worse. Acts 19 as a whole is an example of the opposition to be anticipated when one takes a public stand for Jesus Christ. It takes endurance to establish and maintain a congregation for the Lord Jesus. By the time Revelation 2 was written, the Ephesian church still had good, solid doctrine but had lost the fervor of its first love and needed to repent. Not only the church leadership but the members of the church needed endurance to keep their love fresh.

B. To build our individual spiritual strength and self-discipline – to become more like Christ

Someone who trains seriously with weights will tell you that you need to build "reps" (repetitions) to strengthen your muscles. If you are seeking to memorize Scripture (or anything else, for that matter) you need repetitive study unless you have a most unusually retentive memory. To perform the necessary repetitions requires endurance.

Hebrews 12, which follows right after the great series of examples of faith (both of heroes who triumphed in their signature struggles on earth and those who had the courage to die for the truth), is a chapter based on the concept of endurance. I emphasize the occurrence of the word to make it easier to perceive.

> *Therefore we also, since we are surrounded by so great a cloud of witnesses, let us lay aside every weight, and the sin which so easily ensnares us, and let us run with **endurance** the race that is set before us.* Hebrews 12:1
> *looking unto Jesus, the author and finisher of our faith, who for the joy that was set before Him **endured** the cross, despising the shame, and has sat down at the right hand of the throne of God.* Hebrews 12:2
> *For consider Him who **endured** such hostility from sinners against Himself, lest you become weary and discouraged in your souls.* Hebrews 12:3
> *If you **endure** chastening, God deals with you as with sons; for what son is there whom a father does not chasten?* Hebrews 12:7

This presentation of these verses looks somewhat disjointed but it makes visible the emphasis on endurance in this chapter.

The first image in Hebrews 12:1 is that of a runner. In competition, nobody with any sense would wear a weight vest if trying to win a race then and there. 1 Corinthians 9:24. In this respect there is no difference between a sprinter and a long-distance runner – nobody runs with extra weight if one is running to win. As Christians we are to run our course to succeed in making a pure witness for Jesus Christ, whether successful in earthly terms or not. To take a historical example, Luther and Tyndale were contemporaries. Luther died naturally after translating the Bible into German while Tyndale was executed for exporting Bibles to England in English. Both were faithful to the call of making the Scriptures understandable to people who had no training in Latin. Yet one lived to relative old age and raised a family while the other died a martyr's death. We cannot look at earthly results alone to determine faithfulness. Both of these 16th-century saints ran the race that God assigned them.

THE ENDURANCE OF JESUS CHRIST BEFORE HIS PASSION

Start with Hebrews 5:6-9, referring to Jesus as the eternal High Priest:

> *As He also says in another place: "You are a priest forever according to the order of Melchizedek"; who, in the days of His flesh, when He had offered up prayers and supplications, with vehement cries and tears to Him who was able to save Him from death, and was heard because of His godly fear.* ***Though He was a Son, yet He learned obedience by the things which He suffered.*** *And having been perfected, He became the author of eternal salvation to all who obey Him. (emphasis added to introduce our subject as part of Hebrews 12:2-3 – the quotation is from Psalm 110:4)*

For background, we should go back and consider the relationship between the Father and the Son before the Son took human flesh. Both were present at Creation and in the Garden of Eden. (Genesis 1:26 – note the plurals "us" and "our" – Proverbs 8 personnifies the Son as Wisdom as active at Creation. The Spirit was also present, *"hovering over the face of the waters"* – Genesis 1:2). The Father, Son and Spirit were equal. So the Son had no need to learn to obey the Father because they were always in perfect agreement before Creation. But as part of God's eternal plan the Son voluntarily came to earth to save His people (Matthew 1:21) from their sins and so set aside His equality with His Father. Consider Philippians 2:5-11:

> *Let this mind be in you which was also in Christ Jesus, who, being in the form of God, did not consider it robbery to be equal with God,* [I think the Weymouth version is helpful in the second half of verse 6, so I give its version of verse 6 as an alternative: <u>Although from the beginning He had the nature of God He did not reckon His equality with God a treasure to be tightly grasped</u>] *but made Himself of no reputation, taking the form of a bondservant, and coming in the likeness of men. And being found in appearance as a man, He humbled Himself and became obedient to the point of death, even the death of the cross. Therefore God also has highly exalted Him and given Him the name which is above every name, that at the name of Jesus every knee should bow, of those in heaven, and of those on earth, and of those under the earth, and that every tongue should confess that Jesus Christ is Lord, to the glory of God the Father.*

We must not lose sight of the final exaltation of our risen Lord Jesus, but for purposes of Hebrews 12:2-3 we must focus on His humiliation in descending from heaven to earth. Our Lord Jesus became a baby and depended upon a human mother and adoptive father who were imperfect. (Mary herself needed a Savior – Luke 1:47. In addition, Mary was not in perfect line with the will of Jesus Christ her Son in John 2:1-11 nor in Luke 8:19-21. Mary was a holy woman of God but nevertheless a sinner who needed her Savior.) Through childhood, Jesus grew in knowledge and in all other aspects of human life. Luke 2:40. He obeyed His parents even though He was in essence superior to them. Luke 2:49-51. When He began His public ministry, He was popular with the common people but had repeated conflicts with most of the religious leaders of His time in His earthly body. Jesus Christ twice cleansed the Temple – once near the beginning of His ministry and again near its end. John 2:13-17; Matthew 21:12-13. Many of His earlier disagreements centered around two issues: the Sabbath and His power to forgive sins. (For example, see Matthew 12:1-14 and Mark 2:1-12.) The main point here is that Jesus, being God in human flesh, had to endure contradiction and even insults from those who were vastly inferior to Him. Jesus was accused of blasphemy more than once. John the Baptist, the greatest of all the prophets, had it right when he said that he was not even worthy to untie Jesus' sandal. John 1:27. The centurion who sought healing for his servant recognized Jesus' authority. Matthew 8:5-10. But such honor was rare.

In addition to direct challenges from his inferiors, our Lord Jesus endured a close and personal encounter with Satan. I cannot imagine how repulsive this must have been to the Son of God who is entitled to be worshiped as Isaiah witnessed: *Holy, Holy, Holy.* Isaiah 6:3. Perhaps some clue might be gleaned from the distaste General Eisenhower obviously felt for the Nazi generals who signed the German surrender on May 8, 1945. Try to visualize Churchill negotiating with Hitler. No doubt Churchill would have wanted to throw up. But that is nothing compared to the gulf between our Lord Jesus and Satan. Yet our Lord fasted for 40 days and then endured Satan's temptations as recorded in Matthew 4 and Luke 4. Then Satan tried nothing less than to detach our Lord Jesus from His love for and allegiance to His Father in order to create an unholy alliance to rule the universe or at least the earth. Satan probably hoped that he could induce Jesus to sin as he had Adam. One might speculate that the Greek and Roman myths in which the children overthrew their parents are an echo of Satan's attempt to achieve this in reality. The point for us as we study endurance is that the Lord Jesus endured a direct encounter with Satan. But why?

Our Lord Jesus knew that we too would be fighting either Satan himself or his lesser evil spirits as well as sin more generally. As the Apostle Paul wrote in Ephesians 6:12:

> *For we do not wrestle against flesh and blood, but against principalities, against powers, against the rulers of the darkness of this age, against spiritual hosts of wickedness in the heavenly places.*

And in 2 Corinthians 10:3-5 Paul stated:

> *For though we walk in the flesh, we do not war according to the flesh. For the weapons of our warfare are not carnal but mighty in*

> *God for pulling down strongholds, casting down arguments and every high thing that exalts itself against the knowledge of God, bringing every thought into captivity to the obedience of Christ.*

Peter warned us in 1 Peter 5:8-9:

> *Be sober, be vigilant; because your adversary the devil walks about like a roaring lion, seeking whom he may devour. Resist him, steadfast in the faith, knowing that the same sufferings are experienced by your brotherhood in the world.*

James 4:7 says simply, *"Therefore submit to God. Resist the devil and he will flee from you."*

Our Lord Jesus knew full well that we would be fighting Satan and his allies on earth after He had ascended to heaven. Therefore He endured a repulsive encounter with Satan to show us how such warfare is waged. To Satan's every temptation our Lord Jesus answered with Scripture. So knowledge of Scripture is essential. Then Paul explained the spiritual armor in Ephesians 6:10-18, and also mentions prayer as being critical just as a sentry is critical to military operations of virtually any kind. For our sakes, the Lord Jesus endured the fasting and the encounter with Satan to show us how such warfare is to be fought.

I will end my survey of the life of our Lord Jesus Christ before His passion at this point in order to stick to my subject of endurance. If you want more detail, Alfred Edersheim's *Life and Times of Jesus the Messiah* would be one book well worth reading.

THE SUPREME EXAMPLE OF ENDURANCE: JESUS CHRIST OUR SAVIOR

The great example of endurance in Hebrews 12:2 is Jesus Christ and particularly His suffering on the Cross. Roman crucifixion was designed to kill slowly, painfully and publicly to deter others from the conduct of the condemned. In Jesus' case the placards in the various languages identified Him as King of the Jews. In one sense the statement was true – Jesus of

Nazareth was King of the Jews by lineal descent. The implication of the charge was that Jesus was a rebel against Roman rule, which Pilate knew was false. Pilate knew that Jesus had broken no Roman law. Yet our Lord Jesus endured the ultimate Roman punishment.

This injustice was one aspect of Jesus' bearing our sin. He had been law-abiding in Roman terms but also purely and totally Law-abiding in terms of the Law of God. He fulfilled the types of the Old Testament sacrifices where the innocent animal died in place of the guilty human. Human beings are prone to inflict injustice on one another, so our dear Lord Jesus suffered injustice to Himself to keep us from eternal justice which we deserve. John 15:25, quoting Psalm 69:4.

A closely related aspect of Jesus' sufferings on the Cross was the verbal abuse hurled at Him by his Jewish judges, by the soldiers who whipped Him and even two other crucified prisoners, although one of the prisoners repented before Jesus died. As Matthew describes the first portion of the ridicule and sarcasm by the soldiers:

> *Then the soldiers of the governor took Jesus into the Praetorium and gathered the whole garrison around Him. And they stripped Him and put a scarlet robe on Him. When they had twisted a crown of thorns, they put it on His head, and a reed in His right hand. And they bowed the knee before Him and mocked Him, saying, "Hail, King of the Jews!" Then they spat on Him, and took the reed and struck Him on the head. And when they had mocked Him, they took the robe off Him, put His own clothes on Him, and led Him away to be crucified.* Matthew 27:27-31

As shocking as it sounds, the Scriptures inform us that the Jewish judges who judged Him worthy of death went to Golgotha and mocked Jesus to His face as he was spiked to the Cross.

> *And those who passed by blasphemed Him, wagging their heads and saying, "You who destroy the temple and build it in three days, save Yourself! If You are the Son of God, come down from the cross." Likewise the chief priests also, mocking with the scribes and elders, said, "He saved others; Himself He cannot save. If He is the King of*

> *Israel, let Him now come down from the cross, and we will believe Him. "He trusted in God; let Him deliver Him now if He will have Him; for He said, 'I am the Son of God.'" Even the robbers who were crucified with Him reviled Him with the same thing.* Matthew 27:39-44

> *Reproach has broken my heart, and I am full of heaviness; I looked for someone to take pity, but there was none; and for comforters, but I found none.* Psalm 69:20

Even worse, all this occurred just after the execution squad stripped Jesus naked and gambled for His clothing, as predicted by the Scriptures. Psalm 22:18 fulfilled in John 19:23-24.

The Son of God had always had fellowship with His Father. As Jesus of Nazareth, this had continued through the tremendous, agonizing prayer in the Garden of Gethsemane recorded in John 17. But on the Cross this fellowship was broken and God treated Jesus as His worst enemy in order to spare us, who indeed were His enemies. Romans 5:8-10. Jesus, quoting Psalm 22:1, cried out *"My God, my God, why have You forsaken Me?"* Note that here Jesus does not use the term "Father" to cry out to God while Jesus was bearing the full brunt of the punishment for our sins. Contrast this with the prayer in John 17 and Jesus' final cry of triumph on the Cross when His work of bearing our sins was finished: *"Father, into Your hands I commit My spirit."* Luke 23:46. I cannot know all that Jesus was feeling when He was separated spiritually from His Father, but it must have been more terrible than any merely human grief can be. That, too, is part of what Jesus Christ endured on the Cross.

Another aspect of Jesus' torture on the Cross was the darkness inflicted upon Him as part of the separation from His Father. Mark 15:33. One of Jesus Christ's titles was the Sun of Righteousness. Malachi 4:2. John introduces Jesus as the Light. John 1:9. Was the Light to be snuffed out through the darkness? No, but the darkness had to be endured because outer darkness is part of the punishment for sin. Jude 6. A few brave American pilots endured darkness as a torture inflicted by North Vietnamese captors. Our Lord Jesus endured a darkness more painful even than that because he was and still is the Light. The Resurrection is proof that the Light has overcome the darkness, but we should still remember the darkness as part of what Jesus endured for our sakes.

Jesus endured sleeplessness as a consequence of being tried at night contrary to standing law. There was no break between His arrest at Gethsamane and His Crucifixion at Golgotha. This, too, is part of the punishment for sin. Revelation 14:11.

Thus far I have skirted the purely physical aspects of Jesus' sufferings the night before and on the Cross. These must also be considered at least briefly. Our Lord Jesus sweated blood in interceding for His church in John 17. When He was whipped with a lash loaded with sharp-edged fragments, His skin was shredded to the point where it gave no more protection than a torn leper's coat gave to a leper. Leviticus 13:45. This, too was a step in bearing the total penalty for the sins of many, for the sins of His people (Matthew 20:28 – see also Matthew 1:21). Jesus suffered progressive shock from loss of blood through His entire ordeal – his heart had to beat faster and faster to make up for the increasing loss of blood from the scourging and then the wounds by which He was spiked to the Cross. Jesus was literally shedding His blood for our sins. We have already mentioned the blows to the head when Jesus was crowned with thorns. Isaiah prophesied about Jesus:

> *I gave My back to those who struck Me, And My cheeks to those who plucked out the beard; I did not hide My face from shame and spitting. Isaiah 50:6, fulfilled as noted in Mark 15:19.*

So the prophecy seems to tell us that the cruel soldiers who mocked Jesus also grabbed His beard and yanked some of it out, perhaps with two soldiers pulling from opposite sides of His face at once. No wonder that Isaiah says again that *"so His visage [face] was marred more than any man."* Isaiah 52:14. Such treatment would have ballooned His face until it was almost unrecognizable as a human face. It should shock us that Jesus had to endure this much pain for our sin – we should understand better how grave our sin really is and how important that as believers we put sin within us to death.

And yet there is more pain than I have described yet. The act of spiking Jesus to the cross would have severed nerves that permit human beings to control their hands and feet. This fact should write *finis* to any claim that Jesus did not die. If He had been taken off the Cross alive, He would have been helpless because of the severed nerves, not to mention His other injuries. Also, serum (blood and water) came out of the periocardial sac when the soldier pierced it with a spear. John 19:34, fulfilling Zechariah 12:10 in part. It is quite true that our Lord Jesus endured great physical pain as well as spiritual and emotional anguish, but to climax it all He endured <u>death</u>.

However, we must also realize and give thanks that His sufferings to pay for our sins were complete as His death. Just before His death the Lord Jesus cried out *"It is finished!"* from the Cross. John 19:30. What Jesus meant is that He had completed His final payment of the price for our redemption and had paid the entire penalty for the sins of His people. This is confirmed in Romans 6:9-11:

> *... knowing that Christ, having been raised from the dead, dies no more. Death no longer has dominion over Him. For the death that He died, He died to sin once for all; but the life that He lives, He lives to God. Likewise you also, reckon yourselves to be dead indeed to sin, but alive to God in Christ Jesus our Lord.*

Hebrews 9:25-28 confirms that the sufferings of Jesus Christ have ended:

> *Nor yet that He should offer himself often, as the high priest enters into the holy place every year with blood of others; For then must He often have suffered since the foundation of the world: but now once in the end of the world hath he appeared to put away sin by the sacrifice of Himself. And as it is appointed unto men once to die, but after this the judgment, so Christ was once offered to bear the sins of many; and unto them that look for Him shall He appear the second time without sin unto salvation.*

So we when we contemplate the enormous sufferings of Jesus Christ as part of our own spiritual exercises to build our endurance as commanded in

Hebrews 12:2 (and also to increase our gratitude!) we do need to temper our thinking with the realization that the sufferings of Jesus Christ are over forever.

As a simple summary, we need endurance to be like Jesus Christ.

C. TO USE CHASTENING PROPERLY WE NEED ENDURANCE

Hebrews 12:6-7 tells us that all children of God receive chastening. In the human analogy, this depending on circumstances can range from a verbal rebuke or warning to a serious, painful spanking (but without lasting injury – there is a great difference between a legitimate spanking for correction without injury and brutality designed to degrade and leave long-term injury). For parents bringing up children in the light of Biblical teaching, leaving children without discipline is unthinkable. So much more with our heavenly Father. To illustrate our need for endurance, imagine a horse that stops and rolls over the first time the rider applies a light whip or pulls on the reins. That horse would never finish a task or even plow a field. It would be utterly useless. Yet some people who claim to be believers in Jesus Christ freeze in shock the first time a pastor's sermon steps on their toes or the first time the Holy Spirit begins convicting him or her about a sin that must stop or a new habit that must start. Or the person may take offense from the exhortation of another. Perhaps from a lack of discipline in a person's parental home (if true in one's life) comes a wrong expectation that a new spiritual home will likewise lack discipline. Every child of God, whatever his or her earthly background, needs and receives spiritual chastening. John 15:1-6 is an additional Scripture that teaches about the spiritual discipline of the Father. The presence of parental chastening by the Father is a mark of genuine family membership; its absence is a warning that the person is not yet saved and remains outside the family of God. For a particularly severe statement of this basic truth in circumstances of blatant defiance of God by a believer, see 1 Corinthians 5:1-13. Apparently the person did respond to the discipline and returned to the congregation. 2 Corinthians 2:5-8.

Returning to Hebrews 12:6-7, we are to be exercised by God's chastening. If the physical analogy holds true, that means that we will have to systematically attack the identified sin in order to put it to death in our lives. If we suffer an injury in physical life, we often have to go through an exercise program designed to restore the strength of the weakened part of the body with gradually increasing stress. If our weakness is a lack of Bible study or prayer, we will have to create a new habit and gradually increase our "reps" in order to grow stronger. If we are dealing with the presence of a particular sin, then we must not only stop that particular sin but replace it with something else. On the topic of stealing, the Apostle Paul wrote in Ephesians 4:28, *"Let him who stole steal no longer, but rather let him labor, working with his hands what is good, that he may have something to give him who has need."* Here stealing is to be replaced with work. The greed that triggers stealing is to be replaced by generosity. A man who has been looking at racy images on the Internet will not only have to stop that but replace his former activity with something wholesome. This might be Bible study, prayer, spending more time with his wife if he is married or something else that will help him crowd out the sin to be eliminated. This can be done only through the power of the Holy Spirit, but it must be done. The old Puritan saying is true: <u>either you are killing sin or sin is killing you.</u>

I do not pretend that one's first attempt to put sin to death in one's life as commanded by Romans 8:13 will always be a complete success. There are instances where people have been instantly and miraculously cured of drug or alcohol addiction or of other sins. But sinful habits are often stubborn. God may permit it to be so in order for you to develop strength for future spiritual battles as yet unknown. In one way or another, you will need to develop endurance to grow in the faith.

<u>D. YOU NEED ENDURANCE TO BE A GOOD SOLDIER OF JESUS CHRIST</u>

While even in modern times soldiering is predominantly a male occupation in civic life, this may not be so true in spiritual life. Paul instructed Timothy (and through Timothy the whole Church) that *"You therefore must endure hardship as a good soldier of Jesus Christ."* 2 Timothy 2:3. In civic life, the training methods of the elite units of the Armed Forces are aimed at training the recruit to be able to and minded to endure hardship for the sake of a good cause. If you have seen <u>Band of Brothers</u>, think back to the training runs up the mountain before Company E was shipped to England, even after a heavy meal in one case. These training runs helped develop the tenacity that enabled the 101st Airborne to hold Bastogne until General Patton's relief column arrived and also saved lives within the unit. A purpose of God's discipline is to prepare us for our spiritual calling, whether it be a pastorate, parenthood, or employment in the world with a dual function as an excellent employee and as a witness for Christ Jesus.

E. YOU NEED ENDURANCE TO ENDURE WRONG FOR CHRIST'S SAKE

Suppose that your calling is into a world that on the whole has little appreciation of Christians or of Christianity. Peter writes about such a situation in 1 Peter 2:18-23:

> *Servants, be submissive to your masters with all fear, not only to the good and gentle, but also to the harsh. For this is commendable, if because of conscience toward God one endures grief, suffering wrongfully. For what credit is it if, when you are beaten for your faults, you take it patiently? But when you do good and suffer, if you take it patiently, this is commendable before God. For to this you were called, because Christ also suffered for us, leaving us an example, that you should follow His steps: "Who committed no sin, Nor was deceit found in His mouth"; who, when He was reviled, did not revile in return; when He suffered, He did not threaten, but committed Himself to Him who judges righteously.*

It will take endurance, in this case coupled with self-restraint, to show a reflection of how Jesus Christ bore the ultimate injustice when a boss wants to punish us wrongfully. This Scripture does not forbid making an honest case for our position, but it does forbid retaliation and insults if our case is not accepted.

Peter returns to this theme in 1 Peter 3:16-18:

> ... having a good conscience, that when they defame you as evildoers, those who revile your good conduct in Christ may be ashamed. For it is better, if it is the will of God, to suffer for doing good than for doing evil. For Christ also suffered once for sins, the just for the unjust, that He might bring us to God, being put to death in the flesh but made alive by the Spirit.

We may have to suffer in this life for doing right. It has been said that there were more Christian martyrs in the 20th century than in the first 19 centuries combined. Although only God knows for sure, the number of governments over large populations who turned to mass murder in the 20th century makes this statement appear reasonable. Short of martyrdom, the attitudes of many large employers in the 21st century has turned less friendly in recent years. Just consider the parties and rising dishonesty that have arisen in the business world. Peter said this in 1 Peter 4:3-4:

> For we have spent enough of our past lifetime in doing the will of the Gentiles-when we walked in lewdness, lusts, drunkenness, revelries, drinking parties, and abominable idolatries. In regard to these, they think it strange that you do not run with them in the same flood of dissipation, speaking evil of you.

So we cannot be surprised if our fellow employees slander or insult us because we refuse to share in ungodly and forbidden practices. Paul agrees in Galatians 5:19-21:

> Now the works of the flesh are evident, which are: adultery, fornication, uncleanness, lewdness, idolatry, sorcery, hatred, contentions, jealousies, outbursts of wrath, selfish ambitions, dissensions, heresies, envy, murders, drunkenness, revelries, and the like; of which I tell you beforehand, just as I also told you in time past, that those who practice such things will not inherit the kingdom of God.

When a choice is forced, we must seek the approval of God over the approval of people.

F. YOU NEED ENDURANCE FOR SPIRITUAL JOY, TO OBTAIN GOD'S PROMISES AND TO RECEIVE HEAVENLY REWARDS

Some of you may have experienced "runner's high." For those who have not, this is a feeling of physical and emotional well-being that comes from vigorous exercise. God has designed a healthy human body to enjoy exercise after training. It takes considerable endurance to feel this – you will not feel this at the beginning of a workout. Perhaps this is why some men enjoy hard physical labor and why many male and female athletes are disoriented when they are not in training.

This is a physical analogy to spiritual joy. Let's start with Luke 6:22-23:

> *Blessed are you when men hate you, and when they exclude you and revile you, and cast out your name as evil, for the Son of Man's sake. Rejoice in that day and leap for joy! For indeed your reward is great in heaven, for in like manner their fathers did to the prophets.*

I'm sure these verses seem strange to many of you. They seem strange to me at first reading. I can easily imagine you or myself asking our Lord Jesus in prayer whether He really meant what He said. My first reaction is to pray something like this, "Lord, do you really want me to rejoice to the point of jumping for joy (as if I had just scored the decisive touchdown or basket or pitched the last out of the World Series!) when people isolate me socially and say vicious things about me for Your sake? I would think that popularity would give me a better platform to spread the Gospel." But on more mature reflection I believe that our Lord meant what He said. Our Lord Jesus rarely spoke sarcastically – His habit was straightforward speech. More than that, the witness of history supports a straightforward understanding of His words.

The passage itself mentions the prophets. How popular was Elijah with Ahab or his cronies when Ahab and Jezebel ruled Israel? Review 1 Kings 18 and the following chapters for the answer. What about Elijah's successor

Elisha? A bunch of teenagers chided him over his baldness and paid for their disrespect by being mauled to death by two female bears. 2 Kings 2:23-24. Isaiah was popular with the godly King Hezekiah, but was sawed in half (yes, this was an ancient version of killing by a wood saw – Hebrews 11:37 alludes to this) under the wicked King Manasseh who succeeded Hezekiah (see 2 Kings 21, especially 21:16, for a detailed description). Jeremiah was thrown into a muddy well and left to starve. It was an Ethiopian – not even an Israelite – who insisted on going to Jeremiah's rescue. (Jeremiah 38) Our Lord Jesus summarized the treatment by the nation of Israel of its prophets who came before Him in Matthew 23:31-35:

> *Therefore you are witnesses against yourselves that you are sons of those who murdered the prophets. Fill up, then, the measure of your fathers' guilt. Serpents, brood of vipers! How can you escape the condemnation of hell? Therefore, indeed, I send you prophets, wise men, and scribes: some of them you will kill and crucify, and some of them you will scourge in your synagogues and persecute from city to city, Therefore you are witnesses against yourselves that you are sons of those who murdered the prophets. Fill up, then, the measure of your fathers' guilt. Serpents, brood of vipers! How can you escape the condemnation of hell? Therefore, indeed, I send you prophets, wise men, and scribes: some of them you will kill and crucify, and some of them you will scourge in your synagogues and persecute from city to city, that on you may come all the righteous blood shed on the earth, from the blood of righteous Abel to the blood of Zechariah, son of Berechiah, whom you murdered between the temple and the altar.*

Our Lord condemned the majority of His contemporaries in Israel and warned them that the innocent blood from A to Z – from Abel to Zechariah – would be visited upon them. Indeed the majority was about to kill someone greater than all of these worthy men and women combined – the perfect Son of God, the rightful King of Israel. For purposes of our subject we need to notice the contrast between the prophets and their contemporaries in God's sight. Most of the prophets were hated in the own time, and many were killed. The prophets' enemies often enjoyed the perquisites of power and wealth. But who was rich in the sight of God? Who had treasure in heaven?

Our Lord instructed us to rejoice if we were treated like the ancient prophets for His sake. It is also all too easy to get in trouble for our own sins (for example, 1 Peter 2:20, 3:17). Obviously, it takes spiritual endurance to see beyond human hatred to divine love.

The testimony of later history certainly lines up with the Scriptures looking back at the prophets. History records that all the Apostles with the possible exception of John died violently. In American history, it is hard to find a President more vilified while in office than Abraham Lincoln. William Wilberforce, who pushed England to abolish slavery, was unpopular for most of his career. Christian leaders from Polycarp in the 2nd century (a very old man when he was killed) to the ten Booms in the 20th century and beyond have been killed for their faith. Some Christian leaders who ended their lives naturally, like Wycliffe, had bloodthirsty persecutors on their trail. Wycliffe's body was exhumed and desecrated after his death. So was that of Oliver Cromwell. Times of popularity for Christians and particularly for Christian leaders are relatively rare. Our course is to seek the approval of God and let the chips fall where they may concerning popularity. This takes endurance to shrug off the insults of our contemporaries.

Several churches in Revelation were commended for their endurance. For the Ephesian church, see Revelation 2:3. While the messages to Smyrna and Pergamos do not mention the word endurance, the substance is there. Thyatira was similarly commended in Revelation 2:19, just before the dire warning about Jezebel. In Sardis very few displayed endurance. In Philadephia, perseverance was present and commended (3:10). In Laodicea there was very little endurance; our Lord to this church said, *"As many as I love, I rebuke and chasten. Therefore be zealous and repent."* Revelation 3:19. To all seven churches a promise was extended to those who overcome. Clearly, endurance is essential to the ability to overcome and receive the blessings promised by God.

Consider also Revelation 12:11: *"And they* (the brethren – see verse 10 for the antecedent) *overcame him* (the accuser of the brethren is the antecedent in verse 10 – the accuser of the brethren is one identity of Satan) *by the blood of the Lamb and by the word of their testimony, and they did not love their lives to the death."* So all believers are at perpetual war with Satan until that war is brought to an end by the judgment of Jesus Christ. In terms of present human existence, that war may cost the believer his or her life, just as past wars such as the Civil War or the two Gulf Wars have had deaths. Staying alive in our physical bodies is not the ultimate objective for the believer. Rather, staying faithful to Jesus Christ is the objective. We overcome Satan spiritually and shine in the resurrection by the Blood of the Lamb (which is the payment for our sin) and by our testimony, our witness.

James in James 5:11 says that *"We count them blessed who endure."* In some translations the word "happy" is used. Paul says in Romans 5:3-4 that, *"we also glory in tribulations, knowing that tribulation produces perseverance; and perseverance, character; and character, hope."* Both of these verses link endurance (or perseverance) and joy. How else can we glory in tribulations? We can so glory because we can know that behind the tribulation is the good purpose of God to mold our lives and our characters. *"And we know that all things work together for good to those who love God, who are called according to His purpose."* Romans 8:28. This is as true in the 21st century or in any future centuries that may exist as it was for Paul or for the believers before Christ. Believers of any age can with profit remind one another, *"For you have need of endurance, so that after you have done the will of God, you may receive the promise."* Hebrews 10:36. Our Lord Jesus spoke in the context of the end of the ages, *"But he who endures to the end shall be saved."* Matthew 24:13. It is never that we can earn one iota of our salvation, but His words hark back to the Parable of the Soils, where fruitfulness and endurance is essential to bring forth a crop. Endurance and fruitfulness are the evidence of genuine salvation. **Let us ask God to increase our endurance in line with the challenges we will face. Amen.**

APPENDIX A

THE KINGDOM OF GOD V. THE KINGDOM OF SATAN

Our Lord Jesus said in Luke 10:18, *"I saw Satan fall like lightning from heaven."* I believe that this foreshadows that Satan would be cast down (Revelation 12:7-10). If I understand the symbols correctly, this was done when our Lord Jesus rose from the dead (compare John 20:17) and first ascended to heaven. Satan can no longer enter into the presence of God and accuse us the same way as he accused Job.

More than this, consider the portion of the temptation of Jesus Christ relating to ruling the nations (from a Jewish perspective, the Gentiles). In the main, at Jesus' birth Satan held spiritual sway over the nations. A few Gentiles, such as the Queen of Sheba and Jonah's contemporaries in Nineveh, had believed and worshiped the true God. Matthew 12:41-42; Luke 11:30-32. The Wise Men knew and believed the truth. But in general Satan held sway over the nations. Satan claimed such authority in tempting Jesus with the rulership over the nations, and Jesus did not directly contradict Satan at that moment.

Jesus Christ would indeed be the Light to the Gentiles. Isaiah 11:10, 42:1-6, 49:1-10. But He would not take His rightful place as a vassal of Satan, from a wicked source. Instead of compromising as Satan offered, our Lord Jesus endured the death of the Cross and purchased the nations by His blood from His Father. He then breached Satan's Kingdom over the Gentiles, using first Peter and then Paul to open all-out missionary activity to them. The Apostle John followed, and then generation after generation after all of the Apostles had left the earth. Satan's last-gasp effort to reassert his control over the nations through the AntiChrist will be utterly destroyed by the return of Jesus Christ to the earth.

APPENDIX B

GOD'S REWARDS

Paul speaks of rewards especially to the Corinthian church. Consider 1 Corinthians 3:9-15 where Paul contrasts different types of building materials on the foundation of Jesus Christ:

> *For we are God's fellow workers; you are God's field, you are God's building. According to the grace of God which was given to me, as a wise master builder I have laid the foundation, and another builds on it. But let each one take heed how he builds on it. For no other foundation can anyone lay than that which is laid, which is Jesus Christ. Now if anyone builds on this foundation with gold, silver, precious stones, wood, hay, straw, each one's work will become clear; for the Day will declare it, because it will be revealed by fire; and the fire will test each one's work, of what sort it is. If anyone's work which he has built on it endures, he will receive a reward. If anyone's work is burned, he will suffer loss; but he himself will be saved, yet so as through fire.*

From this passage we can see that salvation is not at issue, but reward or loss is at issue. Paul again instructed the Corinthians about this in 2 Corinthians 5:9-10:

> *Therefore we make it our aim, whether present or absent, to be well pleasing to Him. For we must all appear before the judgment seat*

> *of Christ, that each one may receive the things done in the body, according to what he has done, whether good or bad.*

The first phrase of this passage is again addressed to Christians. Even though we have a common salvation, distinctions will be made accordingly to faithfulness and accomplishment when believers are judged by Christ Jesus, our Master and Lord. Moses *"looked to the reward."* Hebrews 11:26. So rewards should be an incentive for us to be faithful and holy and to achieve what our Lord sets before us. We are also instructed not to permit anyone to take our rewards away. Colossians 2:18; 2 John 8.

Our Lord Jesus taught a clear connection between enduring persecution faithfully and a reward, although no specifics are given. Matthew 5:12; Luke 6:23. Even one who gives someone a cup of cold water will receive a reward. Matthew 10:42 (see also 10:41); Mark 9:41 In some of these cases we cannot be sure whether the rewards are on earth, in heaven or both. In this appendix I have focused on rewards in heaven. I would infer that heavenly reward is what Paul mentions in 1 Corinthians 9:17-18.

The Holy Scriptures speak of two and perhaps three kinds of crowns given as a reward. Paul knew that a "crown of righteousness" was waiting for him after his death. 2 Timothy 4:8. This is given to those who love the appearing (i.e. the Second Coming) of the Lord Jesus Christ. In James 1:12 our Lord's half-brother wrote this:

> *Blessed is the man who endures temptation; for when he has been approved, he will receive the crown of life which the Lord has promised to those who love Him.*

So there is a crown of life for those who love Jesus Christ. Endurance is a part of the qualifications for this crown. Peter in 1 Peter 5:4 writes of a crown of glory that in the context of the passage seems to be limited to pastors, although I would not be certain of this. Needless to say, any crowns or other rewards that we may receive are insignificant compared to the crown of glory of Jesus Christ, which is reserved for Him alone. Hebrews 2:9. But it will still be a blessing to at least have a crown to cast before Him in worship as did the twenty-four elders in Revelation 4:10.

To keep perspective, we should remember that the chief blessing is the common salvation, although rewards have their importance. To describe the common salvation completely would at least take a book in itself and is probable impossible for imperfect human beings. I will mention Isaiah 61:1-3 as one quick summary of the greatness of our salvation regardless of rewards:

> *The Spirit of the Lord God is upon Me, because the Lord has anointed Me to preach good tidings to the poor; He has sent Me to heal the brokenhearted, to proclaim liberty to the captives, and the opening of the prison to those who are bound; to proclaim the acceptable year of the Lord, and the day of vengeance of our God; to comfort all who mourn, to console those who mourn in Zion, to give them beauty for ashes, the oil of joy for mourning, the garment of praise for the spirit of heaviness; that they may be called trees of righteousness, the planting of the Lord, that He may be glorified.*

APPENDIX C

A BRIEF NOTE ON 2 TIMOTHY 2:12-13

In some English translations 2 Timothy 2:12-13 may be confusing. We should start with the teaching of the Lord Jesus in Matthew 10:32-33:

> *Therefore whoever confesses Me before men, him I will also confess before My Father who is in heaven. But whoever denies Me before men, him I will also deny before My Father who is in heaven.*

This passage teaches the necessity of public witness to our loyalty to Jesus Christ. I would understand that denial by Jesus as Judge before the Father is the equivalent of *"I never knew you. Depart from Me, you who practice lawlessness."* Matthew 7:23.

Yet we know that Peter denied our Lord three times and was forgiven. It should also be remembered that Peter had affirmed his faith in Jesus Christ before and after his failure on the night Jesus was arrested. His denials were not characteristic of Peter's total life. We should also recall that Peter's lies concerned whether or not he was a disciple of the Lord Jesus. He never flatly denied His Deity or that He is the Son of God.

Now we need to consider 2 Timothy 2:12-13:

> *If we endure, we shall also reign with Him. If we deny Him, He also will deny us.*
> *If we are faithless, He remains faithful; He cannot deny Himself.*

One immediate point is that endurance is again a condition of reigning with Christ.

Some Scriptures, such as these verses, require spiritual wrestling to understand. So for the rest, I consulted the notes edited by R.C. Sproull, an excellent modern commentator, to the English Standard Bible. I also looked at the commentary of John Gill, an ancient commentator known for his close attention to the Scriptures. I also looked at Strong's Concordance and tried other resources, such as the Matthew Henry commentaries. None of these commentators, nor any others, are infallible. We should not be ashamed to seek help with a passage that causes us trouble so long as we scrutinize any comments (including my own!) as fallible and lacking the full inspiration of Scripture. Having consulted other writers, my explanation is solely my responsibility. I know that I will in terms of rewards or detriments be judged by my Lord Himself for what I write.

What does it mean in this passage to "deny Him"? The most reasonable understanding in the light of all of the Bible is that it means a denial of the essential person of Jesus Christ. It is worse than doctrinal error. It is denying Christ Himself. This explanation matches up with other Scriptures dealing with public confession of faith and for that reason I believe it to be right.

> *... that if you confess with your mouth the Lord Jesus and believe in your heart that God has raised Him from the dead, you will be saved. For with the heart one believes unto righteousness, and with the mouth confession is made unto salvation. Romans 10:9-10*
> [Note: it is commonly understood that the grammatical construction translated as "the Lord Jesus" can and probably should be rendered "Jesus as Lord". Compare 1 Corinthians 15:47 where the Lord Jesus is identified as the "Lord from Heaven."]

> *Therefore I make known to you that no one speaking by the Spirit of God calls Jesus accursed, and no one can say that Jesus is Lord except by the Holy Spirit. 1 Corinthians 12:3*

> *Who is a liar but he who denies that Jesus is the Christ? He is antichrist who denies the Father and the Son. Whoever denies the Son does not have the Father either; he who acknowledges the Son has the Father also. 1 John 2:22-23*

> *By this you know the Spirit of God: Every spirit that confesses that Jesus Christ has come in the flesh is of God, and every spirit that does not confess that Jesus Christ has come in the flesh is not of God. And this is the spirit of the Antichrist, which you have heard was coming, and is now already in the world. 1 John 4:2-3*

I will include 1 John 5:9-12 because I believe that its subject matter is closely related to the previous verses even though it does not expressly deal with public confession. As background for these verses, the Gospels record at least two instances in which the voice of God from heaven validated audibly the claims of the Lord Jesus to be the Son of God (Mark 1:11, 9:7; also Matthew 3:17, 17:5; Luke 3:22, 9:35), in addition to such public proofs as the numerous healings and the resurrection of Lazarus, the brother of Mary and Martha recorded in John 11.

> *If we receive the witness of men, the witness of God is greater; for this is the witness of God which He has testified of His Son. He who believes in the Son of God has the witness in himself; he who does not believe God has made Him a liar, because he has not believed the testimony that God has given of His Son. And this is the testimony: that God has given us eternal life, and this life is in His Son. He who has the Son has life; he who does not have the Son of God does not have life. 1 John 5:9-12*

Some commentators view "faithless" in 2 Timothy 2:13 as representing a momentary failure short of complete apostasy. The Greek interlinear Bible using the Textus Receptus by George Ricker Berry uses "unfaithful" in place of "faithless," which if correct would support this interpretaton. Others leave open the possibility that it should be read as synonymous with the denial of the previous verse, even though the two Greek words are different. In either case our Lord Jesus will always remain true to His own nature and His own words, as John Gill observed. Given His treatment of Peter, I believe that His remaining faithful in the face of our faithlessness means primarily that He will save us despite a temporary failure of our faith such as Peter experienced. Thomas Cranmer in the history of the English Church did also. David's moral fall and restoration are especially pertinent because David was clearly in a covenant relationship with God when he committed his greatest sin involving Uriah and Bathsheba. Our Lord Jesus will not reject one whom He died to redeem. As our Advocate He will never drop a client whom He has taken or lose a case. 1 John 2:1. Neither will God again hold us to account for a sin that Jesus has propitiated. 1 John 2:2. But His Spirit will not permit a redeemed sinner to commit the kind of offense that would of itself consign that person to eternal damnation. Remember that the Lord Jesus will be true to His own words in John 6:37: *"All that the Father gives Me will come to Me, and the one who comes to Me I will by no means cast out."* So once again we come to the conclusion: <u>A true believer will never commit an unpardonable sin. If you have truly come to Christ Jesus and trusted as Lord and Savior, He will bring you home to His heaven.</u>

APPENDIX D

THE PRESERVING POWER OF GOD

Jude introduced his letter as written *"to those who are called, sanctified by God the Father, and preserved in Jesus Christ."* Peter refers to those who are *"kept* (literally *guarded* or *garrisoned*) *by the power of God through faith for salvation ready to be revealed in the last time."* 1 Peter 1:5. Our Lord Jesus promised that *"I will never leave you nor forsake you."* Hebrews 13:5. Perhaps the strongest passage on this subject is Ephesians 1:4-6, which says,

> ... *just as He chose us in Him before the foundation of the world, that we should be holy and without blame before Him, in love having predestined us to adoption as sons by Jesus Christ to Himself, according to the good pleasure of His will, to the praise of the glory of His grace, by which He has made us accepted in the Beloved.*

Unlike us, God is able to visualize a plan of any size all at once. To understand even in part, we often have to reason in sequence what God understands instantly. Logically for our limited brains, the order of events would be (1) God's choice of His people before the foundation of the world; (2) God's predestining His chosen people according to His will and choice; (3) God's initial salvation of His chosen person (a dramatic exanple is the salvation of Paul in Acts 9, which by Paul's testimony was predetermined by God – see Galatians 1:15-16); (4) His spiritual preservation of His chosen ones; and (5) Their final perfection *"to the praise of the glory of His grace."*

The ideas are similar to Romans 8:28-30, which reads,

> *And we know that all things work together for good to those who love God, to those who are the called according to His purpose. For whom He foreknew, He also predestined to be conformed to the image of His Son, that He might be the firstborn among many brethren. Moreover whom He predestined, these He also called; whom He called, these He also justified; and whom He justified, these He also glorified.*

This chain of thought starts with the purpose of God, then predestination, then calling, then justification (meaning the forgiveness of sins and being declared righteous before God) and finally glorification. Greek scholars inform us that every one of the verbs in this passage signifies an act which has already been completed, even the glorification. This clearly implies that true salvation is a "done deal" once it is in force. The fact that we are still alive and that the precise future course of our earthly lives remains unknown to us is not significant. God has made His plan and His plan will stand over any opposition that should arise.

Were the execution of God's plans (including His plan of salvation) contingent on human choice, predictive prophecy would be impossible. If the fulfillment of God's plan for the birth of Jesus were contingent on Mary's response (Luke 1:38), the Holy Spirit could not inspire Isaiah to write, *"Behold, a virgin shall conceive and bear a Son, and you shall call His name Emmanuel."* Isaiah 7:14. Neither could Daniel 9:24-27 have been written, which predicts the time of the Crucifixion, which in turn hinges on the time of the birth of Jesus Christ. Neither could Micah 5:2 have predicted the place of Messiah's birth if the Messiah's mother were unknown to the Holy Spirit hundreds of years before His birth.

If it should be argued that God's sovereign action applies to the Messiah but not to others, Romans 9, 10 and 11 foreclose that argument. To take one example of God's justice without mercy, God raised up Pharaoh for the very purpose of throwing him down and smashing him and his power to bits. Romans 9:17. We also see that the course of life of Esau and of Jacob were determined before either had performed an act on his own. Romans

9:11-13. The salvation of the nation of Israel despite previous rejection is foretold in the last part of Romans 11. The main fulfillment of this is yet future.

Paul in praying for the Philippian church was *"confident of this very thing, that He who has begun a good work in you will complete it until the day of Jesus Christ."* Philippians 1:6

Another clear example of God's initial call and preservation is the Apostle Paul. The risen Christ said to the Ananias who baptized Paul (Acts 9:16), *"For I will show him how many things he must suffer for My name's sake."* Paul had not yet been trained, but Jesus' plans were already fully formed although not fully revealed. Along this same line is Ephesians 2:10, which states that *"For we are His workmanship, created in Christ Jesus for good works, which God prepared beforehand that we should walk in them."* So God has already prepared our good works for us to do. Clearly He will preserve us so that we carry out His plans. He permits both our love for His Son Jesus and remaining sinfulness to express themselves in ways that do not frustrate His designs. We do not become robots. But part of His purpose is our ultimate salvation, and His purpose will be done. The fact that some of His people have fallen badly (David, Samson, Peter for examples) and yet recovered is powerful testimony to His good will and purpose in preserving us forever. Remember that the Good Shepherd was not content to stay with the 99 sheep – He went and found the straying 100th sheep and brought it back to the fold. Matthew 18:12-14; Luke 15:3-7. Matthew 18:14 sums it up, *"It is not the will of your Father Who is in heaven that one of these little ones should perish."*

www.ingramcontent.com/pod-product-compliance
Lightning Source LLC
Chambersburg PA
CBHW070425080426
42450CB00030B/1408